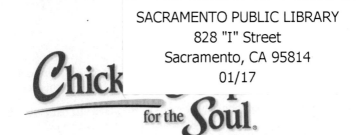

Chick
for the Soul.

D0036521

Chicken Soup for the Soul: Curvy & Confident
101 Inspirational Stories about Loving Yourself and Your Body
Amy Newmark, Supermodel Emme and Natasha Stoynoff

Published by Chicken Soup for the Soul, LLC www.chickensoup.com
Copyright ©2016 by Chicken Soup for the Soul, LLC. All Rights Reserved.

The publisher gratefully acknowledges the many publishers and individuals who granted Chicken Soup for the Soul permission to reprint the cited material.

Front cover photo courtesy of Shinsuke Kishima
Back cover photo courtesy of iStockphoto.com/Salzburg13 (©Salzburg13l)
Interior photo courtesy of iStockphoto.com/JulNichols (©JulNichols)
Interior photo of Amy Newmark courtesy of Susan Morrow at SwickPix
Interior photo of Emme courtesy of Heath Latter

Cover and Interior by Daniel Zaccari

Distributed to the booktrade by Simon & Schuster. SAN: 200-2442

Publisher's Cataloging-In-Publication Data
(Prepared by The Donohue Group, Inc.)

Names: Newmark, Amy, compiler. | Emme, compiler. | Stoynoff, Natasha, compiler.
Title: Chicken Soup for the Soul : curvy & confident : 101 inspirational stories about loving yourself and your body / [compiled by] Amy Newmark, Supermodel Emme, Natasha Stoynoff.
Other Titles: Curvy & confident : 101 inspirational stories about loving yourself and your body | Curvy and confident
Description: [Cos Cob, Connecticut] : Chicken Soup for the Soul, LLC [2016]
Identifiers: LCCN 2016957684 | ISBN 978-1-61159-965-7 (print) | ISBN 978-1-61159-264-1 (ebook)
Subjects: LCSH: Body image in women--Literary collections. | Body image in women--Anecdotes. | Self-esteem in women--Literary collections. | Self-esteem in women--Anecdotes. | Women--Health and hygiene--Literary collections. | Women--Health and hygiene--Anecdotes. | LCGFT: Anecdotes.
Classification: LCC BF697.5.B63 C45 2016 (print) | LCC BF697.5.B63 (ebook) | DDC 306.4/613--dc23

PRINTED IN THE UNITED STATES OF AMERICA
on acid∞free paper

25 24 23 22 21 20 19 18 17 16   01 02 03 04 05 06 07 08 09 10 11

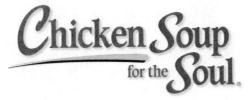

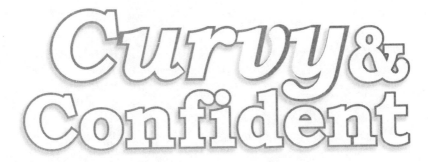

101 Stories about Loving Yourself *and* Your Body

Amy Newmark
Supermodel Emme
Natasha Stoynoff

Chicken Soup for the Soul, LLC
Cos Cob, CT

Changing your life one story at a time®
www.chickensoup.com

Table of Contents

❸

~Sharing the Wisdom~

❹

~Nourishing My Body~

❺

~Living Life with Gusto~

❻

~Warning, Dangerous Curves~

❼

~The Joy of Exercise~

8

~My Miraculous Body~

9

~Larger Size, Larger Life~

10

~Breaking Out of My Comfort Zone~

⑪

~Proud, Pretty, and Powerful~

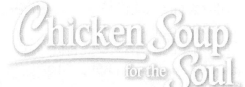

Introduction

When Amy, Natasha, and I first discussed creating *Chicken Soup for the Soul: Curvy & Confident*, we came to the drawing board with a strong, shared belief — that the curvy women of today had a profound need to read body-positive stories, now more than ever.

We could feel the world was at a tipping point when it came to embracing different body types for women, and that we needed to nudge it over the edge.

As one of the world's first plus-size supermodels in the early 1990's, I fought to combat negative perceptions and narrow-minded thinking about women's bodies. I talked until my voice was hoarse, trying to convince people that even if you are larger, curvier, or fleshier, you are still beautiful. The birth of *MODE* magazine in 1997 was a big turning point for millions of women above size 12, and for my career as a model, too. For the first time, we got to see ourselves on the cover of a better fashion magazine in photos created by top stylists, make-up artists, and photographers.

But few retailers understood how to change their mindset from "fat" to "curvy" and this beautiful magazine folded in 2001. We'd been exposed to so many negative messages for so long — in the media, from our families, and even from our own thoughts — that a new, healthier attitude was still difficult to establish.

As a long-time Ambassador for the National Eating Disorders Association (myneda.org), I've seen firsthand how destructive the old way of thinking can be for women of all sizes — large, medium, and small. They can suffer from low self-esteem, which narrows their lives, and eating disorders, which can end them.

Today, I'm happy to see that the world, and our thinking, is progressing — and this book is part of that change.

In early 2016, we saw Mattel issue new versions of Barbie, with different body types, including "curvy." We saw the first plus-size model, Ashley Graham, appear in the *Sports Illustrated* swimsuit issue. She looked gorgeous! Curvy women everywhere felt better about themselves; it gave them hope that a new view of beauty was on the horizon.

Those developments gave Amy, Natasha, and me renewed hope and made us even surer that we were onto something. I think you'll find that this collection of stories continues the conversation in a constructive way. You'll probably react the same way that we did as we read the stories — we laughed, we teared up, and we shared the stories with each other and with our families.

Each of the 101 personal journeys in this book is meant to fortify you and lift you up. And I'm guessing they'll bring back a lot of memories, too. Debra Mayhew's story "Skinny Dipping," for example, brought me back to when I was a teenager and tormented myself when I had to walk to the pool in my bathing suit in front of everyone, including the boys. In the years to follow, I realized that everyone was self-conscious and feeling the same anxiety. Today, swimming is one of my favorite sports and I hate to think about the millions of women who deprive themselves of the pleasure of swimming because they don't want to be seen in a bathing suit.

Having just completed the lecture series at the Metropolitan Museum of Art about beauty throughout the ages in classical sculpture, I loved the theme of the celebrated female nude in Lauren Rossato's "Twenty-Dollar Muse" and James Gemmell's "An Art Perspective." Through James's love and study of art, he questions the dramatic change in the body shape of the female subject in art, and rightly so.

After I read "Cracked Rear View" by Cindi Carver-Futch, I wanted to call her and say, "Go girl!" Cindi's self-deprecating humor and triumph made me laugh, and reinforced my gratitude for my own bodacious booty.

And on a more serious note, I am beyond proud to have a story in this book by my younger sister, Melanie Flint. In "My Journey Back to Me," she talks about her emotional survival at the hands of our misguided and troubled father, who used to weigh her once a week and punish her if she went beyond a certain number on the scale. She lived in terror and learned how to starve herself. I had my own humiliation at the hands of our father regarding my weight, but I didn't know until I read this story what my sister had endured after I left home.

Natasha's story, "Go Ahead, Look at Me," closes out this collection. It's the follow-up to a story of hers that had lain dormant since 2005 and found its voice during the 2016 presidential campaign. After she was flung into the spotlight, Natasha describes how the attacks on her looks by a public figure made her feel, and how she overcame them to find a new confidence.

Each story is unique, but we learn this universal lesson from all of them: We are all perfectly imperfect. And to strive to attain someone's narrow idea of perfection sets us up for failure and a lifetime of unhappiness. Life is too short and precious to waste time doing that. We need to be happy *now*, not in 10 pounds or ten years.

Be. Happy. Now.

When I was a middle schooler, my Physical Education teachers always used me in class to demonstrate whatever new sport or activity we were learning. Being athletic came naturally to me. On the field, in school, on the track, in the pool, I was master. I rowed crew in college and I've always loved using my body for sports.

I see my body as that of an Amazonian. I am feminine and strong. I eat healthy, organic food, I hike and swim every day, I eat exotic chocolate from my "chocolate drawer" when I feel like it, and I keep a positive spirit. With this philosophy, my body has found the right weight for me.

As a mother with a teenage daughter, I am keeper of the body image flame. I fill the fridge with a variety of nutritious and delicious foods and encourage a celebratory relationship with our meals. I express confidence in my body because I know children learn from example, not words, and that they watch everything. We eat when we are hungry, and we stop when we are not hungry anymore. I encourage consistent movement, like after-dinner walks, and I strive to live and teach my daughter balance.

With this book, you will know you are not alone. Instead, you'll have dozens of new friends who have the same problems that you have, who share the same insecurities, and who pass along their best tips and advice to make you curvy *and* confident. I felt like I was away on a retreat with a bunch of great women friends as I read these stories.

I hope these stories give you freedom — freedom from shame, guilt, and body bashing. And I hope they inspire you as they did me and that you turn each page and see a bit of yourself there, as I did. And maybe the negative voice inside of you will be so shocked at our brave storytellers taking belly dancing and posing nude and training for a marathon and wearing a mini-skirt... that it will say to you: *If she can do it, so can I!*

There is no better time to embrace your curvy and confident self than now. This is your body and it is unique. Wake up and shine! Write inspiring quotes on your mirrors with lipstick.

It's goddess time in a serious way. Take care of you and love yourself: The women of the future are depending on it!

~Emme

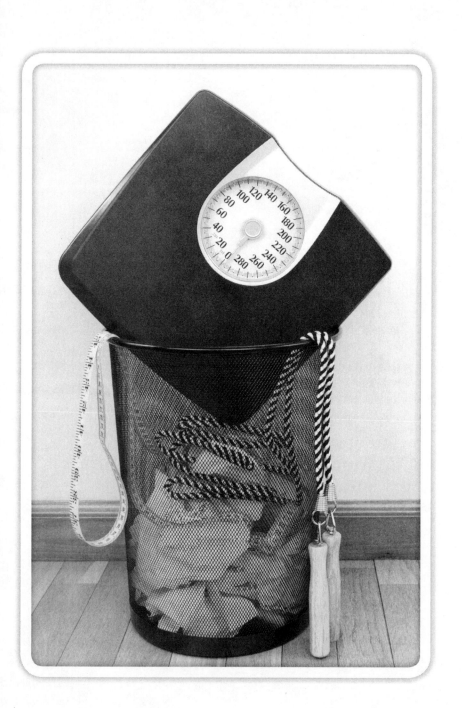

Chapter 1

Curvy & Confident

Look at Me Now

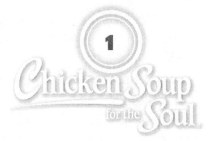

Me, All of Me.

Imperfection is beauty, madness is genius and it's better
to be absolutely ridiculous than absolutely boring.
~Marilyn Monroe

"You're very funny, Sherri. But because you're fat, you'll never play anything but the neighbor or the best friend." After my manager said these words to me, with a pat on my back, I heard her voice and her words ring in my ears for years.

For a long time I was self-conscious about my body. As an actress, I never felt pretty enough or skinny enough to compete with the women I saw on television and on the big screen. But thank goodness for that other voice inside of me, the one that would say: "You can do this girl! You're funny, you're pretty, you're funny..."

Even when I didn't believe in myself, I kept putting in the work — going to acting class and on auditions. I acted "as if" — *as if* I were confidently walking into the casting director's office... *as if* I were going to book the job... *as if* I were a star.

And I let my skills and preparation do the talking for me, instead of the negative voice ringing in my ears.

I listened to other loving, positive words in order to help me overcome the angst, doubt, and unworthiness I felt in this industry. One time, I sat myself in a chair in the middle of a bunch of my friends and had them each say what they thought was special about me that set me apart from others.

From this exercise, I learned that I have a beautiful smile that brings joy to others and that my sense of humor made people forget their own problems. I learned that my knock-knees (which I always hated) made some guys lustful. And I discovered that I am not the sum total of my size 16 clothes or body parts.

My big knees didn't get me a host job on *The View*.

My ample girth didn't secure me a role as the first African American to play the Evil Stepmother in Rodgers and Hammerstein's *Cinderella* on Broadway (and, to be fair, my horrible singing voice didn't either!)

My fleshy arms didn't get me my own show, *Sherri,* on the Lifetime Network (where I got to engage in hot kissing sessions with Malcolm Jamal Warner—yeah baby!)

> *I acted "as if"—as if I were confidently walking into the casting director's office... as if I were going to book the job... as if I were a star.*

My size 9 1/2 feet and my thighs rubbing together didn't land me a top spot on *Dancing with the Stars*.

My round face didn't get me a successful wig line, *Sherri Shepherd NOW*.

In my new NBC comedy, *Trial & Error*, I play a paralegal who suffers from a host of rare disorders that create a lot of humor in the show: short-term memory loss, no tear ducts, facial blindness, foreign accent syndrome, Stendhal's syndrome (fainting around beautiful artwork) and pseudo-bulbar affect (laughing uncontrollably at funerals). She's a very funny character and if me having a double chin somehow helps with this wacky character, then thank you Lord, I accept it.

I walk out the door every day with a bright smile and easy laugh whether I am a size 16 or not. And I've only played the best friend once.

And best of all, when my beautiful son, Jeffrey, rubs my belly and says "Mommy it feels like a Buddha" I laugh. Because the very thing I always hated gives the most precious person in my life joy.

Me. All of me.

~Sherri Shepherd

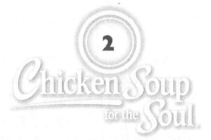

My Journey Back to Me

We have all a better guide in ourselves, if we would
attend to it, than any other person can be.
~Jane Austen

I happily lived in my body until the person I trusted most in the world chipped away at that happiness, replacing it with criticism and shame. Every Sunday during my adolescence, while my brothers were in the kitchen talking and joking and eating a big Sunday lunch, I was in the garage sitting next to the ominous and dreaded stand-up scale, the kind you see at the doctor's office. I always skipped breakfast on Sunday, nervously anticipating my weigh-in. The number needed to be "right" — not one pound more than 123 — according to my father.

My father himself was not slim — he filled the doorway with his tall, thick frame. When he stood behind me as judge and jury, slowly moving the indicator across the numbers on the scale, I held my breath and could feel his own hot breath on my neck.

The moments before the metal arrow slid across the bar and settled on a number were scary. I knew that if the bar moved past the magical number of 123, my father would make me skip lunch and I'd sit alone in my room all afternoon to avoid shaming comments from him. In those moments, I'd hear my stepbrothers laughing and having fun at the kitchen table, wishing I could be thin enough to join them.

I'd starve myself for the next week to avoid the same humiliation the following Sunday. If I'd starved enough, the number would show

120, 121, 122… and I'd get a slap on the butt — the signal that I, too, could go have lunch.

My father did not want a "fat" daughter. The boys in the family were fed well, outfitted with golf clubs and all kinds of balls, boats and guns to keep them entertained and satisfied. I had the scale. The difference in treatment and expectations was striking.

I avoided telling others what was going on at home because I was ashamed. Plus, if I listened too much to others' confusion or anger at why my father was weighing me, or if I believed their positive comments about my body and words telling me that I was beautiful, I might have stood up to my father. And that was not a smart course of action. I needed to be compliant to safely navigate those waters.

So, I kept the weigh-ins a secret. And I began to believe what they meant — that I was not beautiful as me, the way I was; I had to prove my worthiness to myself and others every week.

Needless to say, this was a rocky start toward loving and accepting myself, my body, and everything it provided me.

I spent over a decade, until my mid-twenties, exhibiting acting-out behaviors around food, exercise, and dieting before I realized I needed a new way of looking at myself and my world. That's when I told a dear friend (cocktails were involved, for courage) about Sundays in the garage with my dad and our scale. She listened intently, at times crying, then wrote a name and phone number on a bar napkin and slid it toward me. It was her psychotherapist, whom she said was helping her to change her own life. I took the number and put it away in my wallet, not sure if I would ever make the call.

I was living in New York City at the time, working as a "full-figured model," as we were called in the late 1990's. But the industry did not know what to do with me. I was six feet tall with an athletic build, and while I met the size requirement to be "full-figured," I didn't have "the look" that the clients expected a full-figured model to have.

Even in the plus-size industry, I didn't make the grade. I couldn't figure out where I belonged, what was wrong with me, and how I could fix myself.

Months later, I still had the phone number of the psychotherapist safely tucked away. I wondered if she would make me stand up to my father and call him out on his inappropriate behavior. That still didn't feel like an option for me. The most progress I'd made so far in dealing with him was to hang up on him, slamming the phone down when he upset me. But even that, I didn't do well. I'd feel a rush of self-power in that instant, and then a day of guilt, followed by a half-hearted apology to him to ensure I wouldn't be given the silent treatment for a month.

> *It wasn't my own voice saying those hurtful things about me, it was* **his.**

The familiar and destructive cycle with my father continued for a few more months until one day, I'd had enough. I was finished hating myself and feeling shame and not knowing why. Enough was enough. That day, after one year of carrying her number around with me, I called the therapist.

This wise, kind and persistent woman gently yet firmly guided me through the minefields of misguided beliefs and internalized criticisms I had accumulated and adopted throughout my life. And, shockingly, I came to realize that I didn't actually *believe* the criticisms I'd berated myself with all those years — it wasn't my own voice saying those hurtful things about me, it was *his.*

And so, I began the process of re-recording my own thoughts, opinions and beliefs into my mind, heart and soul. Those realizations propelled my journey toward appreciating myself and having confidence in my true voice and place in any given room or at any table.

In the fifteen years since then, I have realized many dreams. I am married to my true love; I am a mother to three show-stopping kiddos; I have a thriving psychotherapy practice; I have a body that works hard for me and does everything I ask of it; and I have loving and supportive friendships in my life.

We are all worthy of living a great life. And it has nothing to do with the number on a scale, but the plus-size love for ourselves and others in our hearts.

~Melanie E. Flint

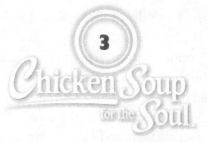

A Confident Triumph

With confidence, you have won before
you have started.
~Marcus Garvey

It was freshman year and my friend Kathy and I were considering pledging for a sorority. Pledge season was full of the usual array of festivities. Throughout Week One, you could sample the various houses at their parties, meeting the sisters and getting a sense of the atmosphere and unique personalities. At the end of the night, if you were interested, you left your card letting them know you wanted to pledge with them. During Week Two the sororities and fraternities got together for combined parties inviting their choices among the potential pledges.

Surprisingly, Kathy chose one of the most elite and highly sought after sororities. It didn't seem like a good fit to me, but she was insistent. I didn't want her to be disappointed but I was doubtful they would choose her. She was just not their type.

Kathy wasn't your stereotypical sorority girl. She was studious. She was kind. She was fashion conscious but she wasn't runway thin by a long shot. She was voluptuously curvy. Unfortunately she was in an environment where curvy was not "in."

Kathy was beautiful inside and out. I just didn't think she was choosing a crowd that could see that.

So we were pleasantly surprised when we both received invitations for the combined party of her chosen sorority and its associated fraternity. I was still skeptical, but I was happy for her.

"Who's your date?" she asked excitedly.

"My date?"

"From the fraternity. Who is the date on your invitation? I hope it's as good as mine. I hit the jackpot. I got Preston."

There was no fraternity brother listed on my invitation. I was concerned. Was it an oversight? Was I second string?

Later I learned the truth, and it was far more sinister. It turned out only some of us were selected for "dates." These chosen few were part of what the fraternity ominously called their Ghoul Pool, an annual tradition.

"I have a date with the cutest, most popular guy on campus. I have the opportunity to show him what a cool and interesting person I am."

The Ghoul Pool was a contest whereby each brother paid his fee and invited the most "ghoulish" date he could find, hoping to be voted the winner and collect the spoils.

I didn't want to hurt Kathy's feelings by telling her, but I didn't want her to walk into such a cruel trap. I debated for days about how to circumvent the party.

Finally on the day of the big event, as she was tearing through her wardrobe to pick just the right ensemble, I told her what I knew. I suggested we skip the party and go to the movies. But she would not be swayed. Despite hearing about the set-up she was determined to go to the party with her date.

I begged her not to go, fearing the night would end in tears. But she insisted. She said she was going to make the most of this date with Preston.

"I have a date with the cutest, most popular guy on campus. I have the opportunity to show him what a cool and interesting person I am," she declared confidently.

So I went with Kathy, fully expecting to have to pick up the pieces by night's end.

At the party, groups of people whispered in corners about "the contest." Throughout the night I heard random comments about the various contestants. Toward the end of the evening I saw Preston being high-fived and congratulated. Apparently, thanks to Kathy, he had won the Ghoul Pool.

I kept watching Kathy, waiting to step in to do damage control if need be. But she seemed to be having a great time. I don't know if she overheard any of the comments about the contest, but if she did, they didn't seem to detract from her enjoyment of the party. At the end of the night, as we were about to leave, Kathy reached up and gave Preston a peck on the cheek. The crowd clapped and whistled.

Kathy and I never spoke about it again. Neither of us pursued pledging that year. Over time, we drifted apart as many friends do.

Years later, one bright spring morning I was headed to Starbucks on my way to a job interview and I ran into Kathy waiting outside the café. We exchanged pleasantries and I congratulated her on her beautiful wedding band and obvious pregnancy. She was glowing, as the cliché goes.

As I was about to make my way toward the door a handsome man came out holding two coffees.

"You remember Preston, don't you?" she chirped.

He smiled broadly, put his arm around Kathy and handed her a caramel macchiato.

~Donna L. Roberts

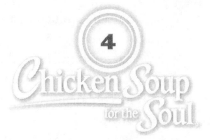

Role Model

The most revolutionary thing you can do
is love your body.
~Author Unknown

I wasn't a skinny kid, but that didn't stop me from dreaming of being a fashion model when I grew up. I used to admire my mother's modeling pictures — Mom was a thin, Twiggy-type model during that era — and dream "what if" and "one day" for myself.

Years later, as a young woman, I stumbled upon an ad looking for plus-size models for a fashion show at a nearby department store. I took a leap and went.

I wore clothes I never thought I'd wear and strutted up and down the center aisle to entice shoppers. It was amazing. My dream became a reality and I told myself: "You can do this!"

I joined a plus-size modeling agency and pursued the passion I had since I was a young girl. I never realized it would have an effect on anyone outside of myself until one day, when I was doing a photo shoot at the beach, I saw a young, plus-size girl watching from the sidelines.

She turned to her mom, excited: "Mommy, I can be a plus-size model!"

It was then that I realized my confidence in my size showed others that they, too, could be confident and do whatever they desired to do in life.

Being plus-size doesn't mean embracing an unhealthy lifestyle. It means the opposite: loving yourself so much that you want the best for you and your body. I've participated in 5K races, danced, traveled the world — I've *lived*. I've dated someone who had never dated a plus-size woman before.

> **Confidence has no size.**

With confidence, you can do anything and go anywhere.

I've been a size 26 and I've been a size 16 and through the sizes I learned how to love myself and take beautiful pictures even at my heaviest.

Today, I still have a role in the plus-size community sharing my story and the stories of others. I write for a plus-size magazine and our motto is: "thrive in your curves."

I tell women at events that you have to learn to love yourself at size 22, because the feelings inside do not just change once you're a size 2.

Confidence has no size.

~Tamara Paylor

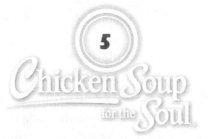

Big Feet in a Small Town

You have brains in your head. You have feet in
your shoes. You can steer yourself any
direction you choose.
~Dr. Seuss

Mr. Winter's voice boomed across the store as I hurried to put my shoes back on. "We don't carry those in size 10. In fact, we don't carry any size 10 shoes for young ladies."

My head sunk lower as a warm flush crawled across my face. My fun trip to the store with my girlfriends to try on new saddle shoes was no longer fun.

Later, when I complained to my parents about the size of my feet, they told me that my feet were doing their job, supporting my body.

"Besides, a nice tall girl like you would look ridiculous with tiny little feet," my father added.

The good thing about growing up in a small town is that you get a lot of feedback. The bad thing about growing up in a small town is that you get a lot of feedback. Neighbors, friends, church folks, even grocery clerks knew my family, and knew that I was the second child, taller and broader than my older sister, and had big feet. What I thought were personal details were topics open for discussion.

On one annual trip to the doctor in the seventh grade, I was measured at 5'8". I overheard Dr. Ostler speak in low tones to my mother in the hall.

"They make a pill to inhibit growth."

I bristled. Hadn't I learned in school that girls were usually taller than boys at my age? This was okay with me as long as they would catch up in the future when I might care, maybe someday *far* in the future.

Mom and I stepped out of the medical office into the hot and humid sunshine.

"What's up?" I asked.

"The doctor says we need to keep an eye on your height and that we can give you a stop-growing pill, if we want to."

> *Our church taught me that my "body was a temple," which meant I was required not only to take care of it, but also to appreciate it.*

"Oh," I frowned. "Can we go get ice cream?"

She nodded and we both shrugged it off, heading to the drugstore across the street for my hand-scooped treat. The subject never came up again.

People described me as "a big-boned girl." My stature came in handy for winning hundreds of "king of the raft" games and rowing my boat down the canal and across Little Lake Jackson. Roughhousing on the sand piles in our yard, I won many "king of the mountain" games, which were loads of fun. And I could see perfectly at the Fourth of July, Veterans Day, and Christmas parades downtown while my friends had to peek around the people standing in front of them.

If I ever compared myself to others, my parents were quick to repeat all the clichés ever known. I grew up with "beauty is as beauty does" and "beauty is only skin deep." Our church taught me that my "body was a temple," which meant I was required not only to take care of it, but also to appreciate it.

At our swim meets, I was the long-distance swimmer for the team. At the end of the season, when my name was called for being the "Most Improved," my heart sank in disappointment — until I heard my family cheering as if it were an Olympic medal. That trophy turned into one of my prized possessions.

My Granny Gert lived next door and sewed most of my clothes. I was happy to have handmade clothes that fit, unlike those from the shops downtown, which had to be altered. I felt lucky to be able to select my own colors and fabrics.

Dad grumbled that I wasted electricity when I held the refrigerator door open searching for after-school snacks. It occurred to me years later that what he was really grumbling about was my chubby, pre-adolescent hands reaching in for more calorie-laden treats, but he didn't know how to address it.

Mom probably worried every year when I watched the Miss America pageant and disappeared into the bathroom afterward to look myself over in the mirror. She made a point to stop whatever she was doing to talk during the commercials. She called the show "entertainment" and held a low opinion of contests designed to judge a person primarily on her outer beauty.

Driving home from town one sunny day, Mom pointed to an elderly woman trudging down the sidewalk. Her back was bent forward, almost parallel to the ground, and I thought she looked grotesque. Mom stopped the car right in the middle of the road and looked straight at me.

"I want you to understand that if you don't stand up straight, you'll look like that someday," she said, which scared me.

So I always stood up straight, but I also always stood out. I thank my physical stature for making me aware of the differences between what people said and their hidden inner thoughts. Someone might ask, "Oh, you're in what grade now? How nice!" while they're thinking, "My gosh, she must be the tallest girl in her entire class." My intuition and people skills flourished as I grew.

Back when I was, in fact, the tallest girl in my sixth grade class and covered with miserable welts and scabs from mosquito bites, a "friend," Shelby, cornered me on the playground underneath the shade trees. She told me every single thing she didn't like about my appearance, starting with my skin's response to insect bites. In shock, I stood there and listened to her angry observations about me and my body—I was too tall, my shoulders too wide, my wrists and ankles too thick, and on and on. I am not sure how I responded but I will always remember feeling alone, horrified, and defenseless.

After school I told my mother what happened. She sat me down and told me that people were going to be jealous of who I was and what I could do because they felt bad about themselves. She said their opinions were more about who they were than about me, and she repeated a quote to me, which I wrote down. It's from "Desiderata" by Max Ehrmann: "If you compare yourself to others, you may become vain and bitter; for always there will be greater and lesser persons than yourself."

I began adding meaningful quotes to my journal and practiced my skills of empathic listening, unconditional understanding and acceptance of others. Later, I graduated with college degrees in psychology and counseling for a lifetime career of helping dysfunctional students and families.

Ironically, in my sixties now, my feet have grown into a size 11. I've been told they will grow even longer as the years go by. But my life has also grown and is filled with love, family, and friends.

And I believe life will grow even fuller as the years go by.

~Wendy Keppley

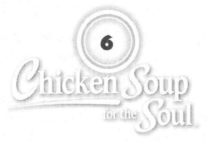

Journey Out of Hiding

Never be bullied into silence. Never allow yourself to
be made a victim. Accept no one's definition of your
life, but define yourself.
~Harvey Fierstein

I was fourteen when I went into hiding. I had been wearing black dress shorts and lace-up black boots, a look I'd seen in a magazine. I thought I looked good, until a friend told me what a boy had said. "He thought you looked nice, except your legs."

That did it. I'd always been insecure about my legs and now I knew it was true. I really did have fat legs — they were too wide, too short and too rounded, just as I feared.

For years after that I only wore loose-fitting pants or long dresses, even in summer, even at the beach. I even swam in jeans.

I tried dieting, cut out soda, and even became a vegetarian in an effort to slim down my legs. Nothing worked. These were the legs I was given.

After college, I decided to try running. I lived with my parents in the country, which was perfect for me — no one would see me. My first run was awful. I was slow and breathless in less than a mile, and I felt like an out-of-shape failure. I wanted to give up, but a friend told me that anything could become a habit after three months. I decided to work out consistently for at least three months. And although the gym intimidated me, I signed up at one so that bad weather wouldn't stop me.

The first day at the gym, I was worried I'd look foolish trying to figure out the machines and worse yet, trying to run. But no one seemed to be paying attention to me. The more I went, the more I realized that other newcomers were there too, starting their own exercise programs and unsure how to use the equipment. I began to feel comfortable at the gym.

I started going three to four days a week, always on the treadmill, mostly walking with just a little running. Gradually, I added more until I was running more than walking. Eventually, I was running for about forty minutes. I went from hating running to loving it, craving it even. I ran five or six days a week and started increasing my distances. The three-month plan had worked for me and my legs were getting stronger.

I only wore loose-fitting pants or long dresses, even in summer, even at the beach. I even swam in jeans.

One day, an instructor running next to me on the treadmill suggested I try her class. A class? My mind raced with excuses: I imagined perfectly toned people looking at me and wondering what I was doing there. I wouldn't know the exercises and I'd look silly. But she was so encouraging that I told her I'd go, telling myself I'd stay in the back of the class so no one could see me.

After trying it however, I felt energized. Within weeks, I was at the front of the class and the instructor was asking me to demonstrate moves. Months later, my instructor friend suggested I apply for an instructor position at the gym.

"Me, teaching? In front of people?"

There was no hiding the shape of my legs in front of a class. But now, having been at the gym for some time, I'd seen all types of bodies and realized that all shapes and sizes were beautiful.

I applied and got the job! I went from hiding my legs to showing them off in tight Spandex in front of a whole class!

Now, I am thankful for my strong legs that power me up hills on my runs, enable me to do squats, and help me hold a pose longer. I wear shorts, capris, yoga pants, skinny jeans, and even a bikini!

I still teach fitness, and I love when beginners come to my classes. I look forward to helping them find reasons to continue — like having more energy, increasing strength and balance, and improving their mood.

I hope they realize that the bodies they have are beautiful, one of a kind. And they should never feel like they have to hide.

~Rebecca Eicksteadt

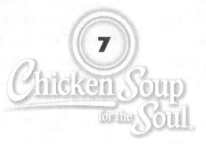

This, But Also More Than This

Is fat really the worst thing a human being can be?
Is fat worse than vindictive, jealous, shallow, vain,
boring, evil, or cruel? Not to me.
~J.K. Rowling

When I was seventeen years old, some guys from my high school mooed at me. I was walking along the side of the road and they hung out the windows of their car as they drove by me and mooed. I was about 25 pounds overweight, and yes, high school guys can be judgmental, arrogant idiots. But being compared to livestock solidified everything I believed about my teenage self at that time — that my looks and my weight were what mattered most to people.

It didn't help that on that particular spring day I was out walking as part of a new resolution to lose weight. I'd gained some after my parents told me we were moving to California the previous summer. During the months before the move, we packed up our house and relocated to a small apartment and I'd quit swimming competitively to spend more time with my friends before we left. I was sad, angry and scared about moving, and part of that manifested itself as weight gain. But once I was in California I had plenty of time to "work on myself." Walking, swimming, and eventually running were part of this new regime. Until those guys mooed at me.

I have been fighting back against that moment of bovine shame ever since.

Why does it matter how much I weigh or what I look like? Sometimes I think trying to lose weight is just a way of giving in to the superficial insanity that keeps women focused on the number on the scale instead of the number of ways they can change the world.

But for some reason, I couldn't forget that moo. There I was, happy that I was following through on my new fitness resolution and instead I was subjected to that awful moment of shame. I went from feeling optimistic to figuring out the fastest, least public way to get back to my house to hide. It's taken nearly three decades to understand that while I was (and still am) overweight, I was also a successful student, a hard-working swimmer, a good singer, a caring friend, an enthusiastic dancer, an avid reader, and a bunch of other things that "moo" tried to obliterate.

When I decided to write a novel a couple of years ago, I knew that my heroine, Maggie, would be overweight.

When I decided to write a novel a couple of years ago, I knew that my heroine, Maggie, would be overweight. I also knew I wasn't going to write a story about her weight or her *losing* weight. I wanted to tell a story about a young woman who is heavy, but realizes that's not all she is. That was the story I needed to hear when *I* was seventeen years old.

Last year that book was published. The thought of people reading about Maggie, who in many ways is the teenage girl I wish I'd been, made me feel vulnerable and elated and ashamed and anxious, just like I did when I was seventeen.

But because of Maggie, I came to understand that I didn't need to write her story to exorcise the demons of getting mooed at; I needed to write her story to figure out what getting mooed at had come to mean to me. And I did.

This is the power of telling our stories, of making ourselves vulnerable in them and to them. Writing about Maggie helped me see that my body is a part of the package, not the whole thing. It helped me see I have talents and abilities and even flaws that have nothing to do with the number on the scale. And it helped me see that a woman with curves and substance can be the heroine of her own story. It might have taken me thirty years to figure this out, but it's been well worth the wait.

~Kris Dinnison

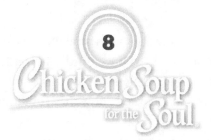

Dancing Away My Insecurities

The dance is over, the applause subsided, but the joy and feeling will stay with you forever.
~W.M. Tory

All eyes were on me as the conversation from the other moms quieted down. Someone had just asked, "Are you going to join us?"

"Yeah, you should dance with us," another encouraged.

I was waiting for my daughter's dance class to finish while the other moms got ready for their adult dance class.

"Nah," I shook my head and smiled politely. "I don't think so."

But the truth was — I wanted to. I'd watched these moms from the sidelines through the years, dancing and laughing together and getting exercise, and it looked like fun. The thing is, I didn't have a dancer's body. I didn't even know if I could dance.

"Why don't you try?" my husband said to me one night, as I stared at my body in the mirror. I think he was reading my mind. "You'll never know if you don't try," he said.

So I signed up for ballet, for the first time in my life.

At my first class, I wondered if I could even get myself off the ground. I was the biggest woman in the room. And to make matters worse, the walls were covered in mirrors. Seeing myself in those mirrors reinforced how ridiculous and horrible I looked. *What did the others think of me?*

The instructor started us with stretches and then moved on to basic ballet positions: first, second, third. My feet followed. So far, so good. Then came some simple steps and soon my feet were moving with the music. Maybe not exactly how they should have been moving, but they were moving.

"Great job tonight, everyone," the instructor said as she clapped her hands. "See you all next week."

I had officially survived that first night, and no one had made comments about my size. So I kept going each week. The instructor moved on to harder steps. Ballet wasn't easy; my muscles were sore and my legs didn't know what they were doing. I still didn't know if it was for me, but I persevered.

> *"I did it! I may not be the most graceful dancer, but I've learned ballet!"*

After a while, I forgot about the mirrors. The steps continued to get more difficult, but I practiced at home with my daughters and we had fun together.

One night at class we were twirling, stepping this way and that, and my legs were getting a great workout. I was keeping up and my feet were doing what they were supposed to do. Later, I realized something surprising. My legs weren't sore anymore.

I saw a difference in the way I carried myself, too. I was stronger. And my muscles weren't the only part of me that had been strengthened. "I don't care how ridiculous others think I look dancing," I told my husband with my new confidence. "I did it! I may not be the most graceful dancer, but I've learned ballet!"

Not long after that, I was shoe shopping and found a pair of tap shoes for three dollars. I hadn't signed up for tap because I didn't think my body could bounce in that way, but when I saw the shoes in my size, I grabbed them from the shelf.

At my next ballet class, I walked in with tap shoes. "Guess what?" I said to the instructor, "next year I'm taking tap, too!"

She looked at me. "Nope. You're doing tap *this* year."

My jaw dropped.

"The recital is in four weeks," she said. "You're a quick learner. You've got this."

And I did. On recital night, I took the stage, threw myself into the air, and danced!

~Jennifer Sommerfelt

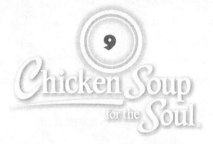

Shape Shifting

Successful people have fear, successful people have doubts, and successful people have worries. They just don't let these feelings stop them.
~T. Harv Eker

It was the morning of my first big photo shoot as a plus-size model and I was excited — and hungry! On the way to the location, I picked up a big box of chocolate and cinnamon rugelach from my favorite bakery for everyone to nosh on as we worked, then wondered if they would all say, "Of course the plus-size model would bring in something fattening to eat!"

I wouldn't care if they did. I was in such a great mood that nothing could bring me down.

My recent career after studying on a full rowing scholarship at Syracuse University was as a local reporter for NBC in Arizona. Then, at age twenty-six, I transplanted to New York to embark on a new career as a plus-size fashion model with Ford Models. I loved my new vocation because I enjoyed exploring what we considered "beautiful" in our culture and other cultures, and why. As a plus-size model, I would be challenging and expanding society's definition of "beauty."

I arrived early at the West Side loft rented for the shoot to find a crew of ten people already prepping — make-up artists, hair stylists, two wardrobe stylists, and various assistants. The only ones who hadn't arrived yet were the photographer and his assistants.

The room was abuzz with activity. We were photographing an ad for blue jeans that day. It would be one of the first full-figured ads to be published in major magazines and on billboards. It was a big deal, and I was the model the client chose!

I was about to earn more money in one day than I usually made in a month. But it wasn't about the money. I could feel something great was going to happen. We were on the verge of a new way of looking at women, we were nurturing a change in attitude about body shapes, and this shoot would symbolize it.

Enter the photographer, who has worked with the biggest publishers and fashion magazines in the world: *Vogue, Elle, Harper's Magazine, Marie Claire*, and *Cosmopolitan*. I was beyond thrilled that I was going to be in front of his lens that day. Except, he wasn't quite what any of us expected. He showed up to the loft looking dirty and disheveled, and seemingly drunk (or hungover?) from the night before.

> *"I am not shooting this fatty!" he yelled.*

Barely giving others a nod, he strode to the back of the loft where I was being made up, my hair in Velcro rollers, and looked around.

"Where's the model?" he asked everyone, and no one in particular.

We all looked at each other, wondering if he had bad eyesight or something. I was sitting right there, three feet away from him. I raised my hand slowly.

"Hi, I'm Emme. Nice to meet you."

The photographer looked at me blankly, and then his whole face pinched as he grew horrified.

"I am not shooting this fatty!" he yelled, and stormed across the room and out the door, slamming it.

We all froze and no one said a word. A minute later, I could feel someone expertly place tissues under my eyes — it was the make-up artist and her assistant, worried I'd start crying and ruin their hour and a half of careful make-up application.

They didn't have to worry; I wasn't upset, I was angry! How dare he speak to me, or anyone, that way? I got on the phone with my agent and explained the situation, telling her I wanted to leave.

"No, you have to stay! He'll be back. No one turns down a

commercial job like this if they want to work in New York."

Over the next hour, everyone took turns apologizing to me for the photographer's rude behavior. I just wanted to leave; I didn't want to face that idiot again. But as my agent predicted, he did return… four hours later — angry and pissed off to be there, too. He didn't say a word to anyone, especially not to me, as he prepped his equipment for the shoot, insisting he'd "only shoot the fatty" right where he was already positioned. He refused to budge an inch.

I wasn't so thrilled anymore to be in front of this guy's lens, but there I went. The photographer walked up to me, placed his hands on the neckline of my shirt as if he was about to choke me, and proceeded to sloppily stretch out the neckline until it fell around my shoulders.

"If I'm going to shoot you," he sneered, "I'm going to shoot you *sexy*."

"Well," I replied, "if you're going to act like this, then let's get this over and done with."

Somehow, we made it through the rest of the workday and created some great photos and the campaign was a success.

Fast-forward five years, to 1994: I'd been featured as one of *People* magazine's coveted "50 Most Beautiful" that year and my fledgling career had taken off. I was in Miami for a photo shoot and we were set up near a café, when I noticed a familiar face at a nearby table. Flanked by two beautiful women sat that idiot photographer. But now he was clean-shaven, spiffed up, and looking very handsome.

At first, I remembered the horror of his words and felt angry. But then as I stared at him for a few moments, it dawned on me that because of this man and others like him, I fought hard in my career and was determined to never give up. Women have always fought to gain respect and fairness, even if it's with other women, too. That photographer's attitude toward full-figured models, and perhaps women in general, showed me that the road to a new way of thinking about what makes a woman beautiful would not be an easy one. There would be many hurdles. But in those five years since that photo shoot, I'd found my life's purpose — empowering women to be the best they can be. And my work and message were being seen and heard in the fashion industry and all over the world.

I decided that I was meant to face this photographer that day so long ago, when his beliefs and stereotypes about women were at their worst. He represented exactly the kind of thinking I wanted to change.

So now it was time to thank this man who had made my life hell for a day. Because, as actor Dustin Hoffman once said as he accepted an Academy Award, "I want to thank those who kissed me and those who kicked me."

I went up to his table.

"Excuse me, I hope I'm not interrupting you... my name is Emme."

He looked up from his coffee and smiled. "Emme! Yes! Oh, we *have* to work together! I'd really love to shoot you. Congrats on all that you are doing."

I was stunned, and more than a little confused. He obviously recognized me and knew me from my photos, but he didn't seem to remember that I was the model from that day in the loft, or what had happened there. He didn't remember causing me pain on a day that was to be bright and hopeful for me.

"Oh, I'd love that," I replied. "Actually, we did work together one time a few years ago... and I wanted to thank you for that."

He looked puzzled, but he shook my hand and smiled anyway. I left for my photo shoot with a smile on my face, too — knowing that despite one man's limitations, we can all expand our horizons and change our attitudes toward each other.

~Emme

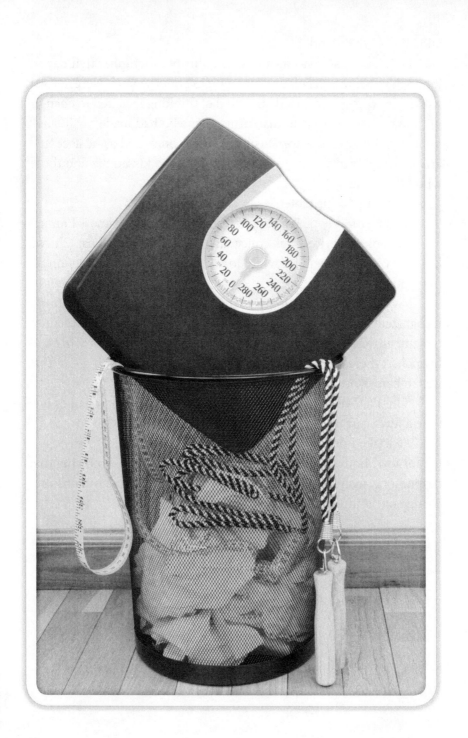

Chapter 2

Curvy & Confident

Real Life, Real Beauty

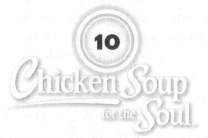

I Believe in Goddesses

A woman in harmony with her spirit is like a river
flowing. She goes where she will without pretense
and arrives at her destination prepared to be
herself, and only herself.
~Maya Angelou

I remember at the tender age of five being sent home from kindergarten for pinching a girl. She was the cutest girl in the class so I decided to show my affection for her by pinching and slapping her chubby bottom. Growing up, my brothers and I often showed affection for each other by punching and slapping each other.

My father addressed this issue by telling me a story. He told me that little girls were special, not at all like little boys. When a little girl was born, he said, all the goddesses in the universe stopped by and touched her forehead. When this happened, a little bit of each goddess went into the girl, and that's what made them so beautiful, kind and loving.

Along with those attributes, though, they also received the power of each goddess. So if you made them mad they could unleash all those goddesses on you. And if that happened, my father warned, you were by yourself and nobody could help you.

"Nobody survives the wrath of a goddess," he warned.

He knew I was fascinated by Greek and Roman mythology and in awe of the power of the deities. I always had nightmares about

being chased and hunted by Diana, goddess of the hunt, or meeting Persephone, queen of the underworld. So the next day, with a big box of chocolate in hand, I apologized profusely to the little girl I had pinched and asked her to please not unleash her goddesses on me. She was very confused, but we soon became fast friends. We became know as the duo, Tubby and Lulu. We were by far the chubbiest and cutest kids in the class and were the stars of every school dance.

Goddesses became a fascination for me, and since my father's story I would look at the girls and women around me and try to spot the goddesses that dwelled in them. I would catch glimpses of Aphrodite, Venus and Juno on a regular basis and to me this totally made sense. How else would you explain stories of women who lifted cars off their kids or confronted men twice their size? This gift that my father bestowed on me enabled me to see women for who they truly were, and began a lifelong love affair with these amazing incredible creatures called women. I wanted to know and understand everything about them.

> *I started looking up pictures of Greek and Roman goddesses. They were curvy and soft, powerful and beautiful.*

I started looking up pictures of Greek and Roman goddesses. They were curvy and soft, powerful and beautiful. I remember drawing them all the time and creating new outfits for them.

I soon knew that I wanted to be a designer and dress these goddesses.

I grew up in the 1960's surrounded by images of Twiggy, and was confused why she was considered beautiful instead of the women who looked like Venus or Aphrodite. I didn't understand why I did not see women in magazines who looked like the women in paintings. In fashion school, my sketches always looked different from the other students — my figures and lines were curvy and round.

When I worked as a designer at Anne Klein, I was part of a team that created the first "full figure" designer line and worked with celebrated women like Camryn Manheim, Rosie O'Donnell and Oprah Winfrey. This was a dream come true for me. Another even better dream come true was creating a groundbreaking fashion brand inspired by Queen

Latifah for VF Corporation.

Women should know that their form represents the form of the goddesses that live within you; your form inspires painters, musicians and designers. When I run across little girls who say they want to be a princess I laugh and look at them and think, "If you only knew that being a princess is way beneath you. Princesses are mere mortals, but you are touched by the goddesses."

So I ask that you find your inner goddesses, nurture them, and unleash them sometimes. Because everyone needs to see who you truly are. Believe in goddesses because they are real.

~Sunil Ramchandani

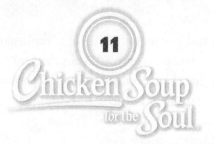

11

Marilyn's Magic

We are all of us stars, and we deserve to twinkle.
~Marilyn Monroe

I was under strict instructions not to touch anything — *especially* not The Dress. But there it was, shimmering and beckoning me from the middle of the room at Christie's, and the security guard had left for the day.

I was working on a magazine cover story in 1999 about the auction of iconic sex symbol Marilyn Monroe's personal items. For the story, I'd interviewed many of her friends and co-stars, including actors Eli Wallach, Celeste Holm, and Lauren Bacall.

The night before the auction, Christie's had given me exclusive and private access to all Monroe's items to look over — exciting things like clothing and make-up, and everyday items like utility bills, pots and pans, and cookbooks.

And… The Dress.

"But don't touch anything!" the guard sternly warned, before he left. I assured him that touching was way, way out of the realm of possibility.

Marilyn Monroe had worn the flesh-colored, skintight, evening sheath the night she breathily sang *Happy Birthday* to President Kennedy at Madison Square Garden in May 1962. Less than three months later, she'd be dead; the following year, so would he.

But with this dress — displayed on a specially constructed, ultra-curvy mannequin nearly forty years later — the magic was still alive.

What magic, you ask? I'm talking about that wordless aura a woman has when she understands and revels in the power and beauty of her female shape.

Many years ago, I had sat next to Marilyn's first husband, Jim Dougherty, at a dinner at the Niagara Falls Film Festival (I got to sleep in the same hotel room she did while shooting the film *Niagara*) and asked him what about her, in person, made her so sensual.

"She believed she was, she *felt* it," he said, describing a memory from the year they lived on Catalina Island when Marilyn, aka Norma Jean, was only seventeen.

"She'd put on a pair of little white shorts and take the dog out for a walk every Saturday at 3 P.M.," said Jim. "The men in the neighborhood made sure to be outside washing their cars or mowing their lawns at that time every week like clockwork, to watch her slowly walk by."

She was no skinny-minny, he assured me. Judging by her films, it looks like she fluctuated up and down the same 20 pounds that a lot of women do, but it didn't seem to bother her so much.

"My husband likes me plump!" she once said of playwright Arthur Miller, when reporters suggested she was getting hefty during the *Some Like it Hot* era and should invest in a good girdle.

I myself was always grateful for Marilyn's ampleness of chest and how she walked proudly with her shoulders pulled back. I, too, was ample in that area, and watching Marilyn in *How to Marry a Millionaire* convinced me to trash my tent-like T-shirts and stop hiding.

In recent years, there has been debate about her actual size. Some fashionistas insist she was a size 16 while others argue that sizing was different back then, and she ranged anywhere from a 4 to a 10, depending on her weight.

Now I looked around me in the auction house. I was alone and surrounded by her clothes. Why not check for size tags? I was pretty brilliant, I thought, until a nearby lime green Pucci blouse and the bulky sweater she wore on the beach in that famous Bert Stern photo proved to be tag-less, and so did a black cocktail dress.

I spied what looked like her driver's license on a pile of books and picked it up:

Height 5'5¾"
Weight 120 pounds

Hmmmm. How was she so curvy? Or did she bat her eyes at the motor vehicle bureau clerk and fill in the form the way the rest of us do — with the weight we intend to be… some day.

I went back to the black cocktail dress and stood in front of the mannequin. With my hands, I measured the width of her waist and then moved my hands to my own middle to compare the two.

> *I'm talking about that wordless aura a woman has when she understands and revels in the power and beauty of her female shape.*

And that's when I discovered firsthand that Marilyn's waist was tiny! She was petite! There was no way Marilyn was a size 16 as we know it today — *ever.*

Not that there's anything wrong with that, because sexiness and beauty, as I was learning, had no size. It was something, as Jim Dougherty described, a woman felt in her flesh and bones and soul. It was in the way she walked and what she knew about herself.

Sexy was an attitude.

But while I was there, it didn't hurt to give my attitude a little boost, right?

The Dress was at the center of the room, and I needed to touch it. Perhaps Marilyn's attitude was still alive in the fibers of the souffle gauze fabric encrusted with graduated rhinestones embroidered in a rosette motif.

I looked around for video cameras and didn't see any, so I made my way toward it. Ten seconds was all I needed to reach out, touch The Dress, let my fingers linger for a moment, then pull my hand back. In that time, a montage of black and white news clips and movie scenes filled my brain — Joe DiMaggio at bat and crowds cheering, Marilyn with her white dress billowing on Lexington Avenue, John Kennedy handsome in the White House, and Marilyn singing "Diamonds Are A Girl's Best Friend."

Ten seconds was all I needed to feel the magic. The next day, I watched as The Dress sold for $1,267,500 — the most ever paid for a single item of personal clothing, even to this day. The new owner of The Dress said it was a steal. And now I see in the news that it's up for auction again.

Unfortunately, a writer's paltry salary doesn't allow for a $2 million dollar dress allowance. Maybe this time, I can buy one of her Le Creuset pots or something.

But no matter. When I left Marilyn's things that night in 1999, I felt like a million bucks. I glided out slowly, with my shoulders back and my hips a-sway more than usual.

I looked like a movie goddess; the night janitor will swear to it.

~Natasha Stoynoff

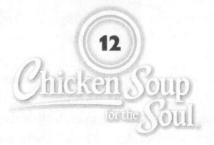

12

A Work of Art

We're telling women that they're plus size. But for me,
I just like to call it curvasexalicious.
~Ashley Graham, plus-size model, on Ellen

I am a fifty-six-year-old male who collects the annual *Sports Illustrated* swimsuit issue. There are twenty-one issues of this classic periodical stacked on the floor of my home office.

Now don't get me wrong, I'm not some kind of dirty old man. I do more than just look at the models. I like to read the sidebars about where the photos were taken, where the crew stayed, where they ate, and what they did while there. Plus, I enjoy the funny ads, like this year's full-page advertisement for Grizzly smokeless tobacco, which boldly states, "You will never date a girl in this magazine." How funny is that?

As for the models themselves, I'm honestly not impressed with a lot of the pictures. I see some of their poses and mumble, "That's stupid." I see some of their sultry, lip-biting expressions, and murmur, "Aw, c'mon. Gimme a break." So I think I'm pretty well grounded.

And so it was. After dinner on Thursday, February 18th, I curled up on my bed with the 2016 swimsuit issue. It was no big deal until I opened the magazine to see a three-page foldout stating, "This body is made to be uncovered." It featured a gorgeous "plus-size" model in a white, two-piece bathing suit.

"What?"

I opened the flap to see that it was an ad for Lane Bryant.

I scratched my head. "What is that doing in the swimsuit issue?"

Undaunted, I continued reading the magazine, turning through full-page ads for typical guy stuff like Edge shaving cream, Breitling watches, and Copenhagen tobacco.

Then I came to two pages explaining the magazine's use of three different covers with three different models: Ronda Rousey, Hailey Clauson, and Ashley Graham. My copy had Hailey Clauson on the cover. I knew that Ronda Rowsey was a famous athlete — but Ashley Graham? Who was she? These same two pages had a picture of Ronda, but not one of Ashley. Thus, I didn't know a thing about her.

> *For the first time in history,* Sports Illustrated *was acknowledging plus-size models in its world-renowned swimsuit issue.*

So from there, I dove into the swimsuit issue, enjoying all the beautiful models and zipping through the ads for light beer, razors, and cologne.

Then I hit page seventy-five and slammed on the brakes. Pages seventy-five, seventy-six, and seventy-seven contained full-page pictures of stunning, plus-size models in golden bikinis. Their ad was for a company called Swimsuits For All. I had never heard of them, but I think I can safely say that I figured out their target customer.

Still, I asked myself "Why is *Sports Illustrated* doing this?"

I continued perusing the issue until I got to page 177. There she was — a striking brunette model named Ashley Graham in a blue, two-piece swimsuit from Lane Bryant.

At first, I furrowed my brow, asking myself "Isn't she a bit... um... big?"

Then it hit me.

For the first time in history, *Sports Illustrated* was acknowledging plus-size models in its world-renowned swimsuit issue. And Ashley was awesome!

YOU GO, *SPORTS ILLUSTRATED*!

The female body is a work of art that is beautiful in all shapes and sizes.

~John M. Scanlan

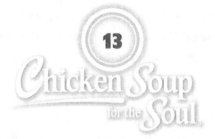

Back to Curvy

Healthy emotions come in all sizes. Healthy minds come in all sizes. And healthy bodies come in all sizes.
~Cheri K. Erdman

The number on the scale plummeted yet again, and with it, my confidence. Yes, you read that right; unlike what society preaches, losing weight isn't always a good thing. Less of ourselves is not necessarily better.

As my curves melted away, my body was sending out the message: "Help!"

I had fully recovered from anorexia over a decade earlier and had learned not to give the scale too much power. I'd even written three books on the topic and given hundreds of talks on embracing a strong, healthy body. Society tells us that being thin makes us happy and successful but I knew this was a big lie. At my thinnest, I was miserable.

And yet, when I unintentionally lost weight due to PTSD, my doctor congratulated me during a yearly exam.

Why was I getting complimented for having a mental illness?

It happened when I had anorexia, too — I received accolades for having a life-threatening psychiatric illness with the highest mortality rate of any mental illness.

Recovering from anorexia, I had learned to think of gaining weight as gaining pounds of happiness. Now, I was in recovery for posttraumatic stress disorder (PTSD) after being raped in my late twenties.

The accompanying depression and anxiety had killed my appetite, the stress had caused havoc on my thyroid disorder and my weight was going down again. Importantly, it wasn't just my body that was shrinking; PTSD itself disintegrates self-esteem.

I wanted my life back. I wanted my curves back.

I come from a family that is naturally thin, so some people might not have considered me curvy in the first place. But I feel that curvy comes in all shapes and sizes because it's not so much a body type as it is a state of mind. To me, curvy means striving for balance, authenticity, and mindfulness. It means listening to and nurturing our bodies and not betraying our souls to look a certain way. It means letting go of shame — something that people battling eating disorders and PTSD know a lot about.

> *To me, curvy means striving for balance, authenticity, and mindfulness.*

I knew from my eating disorder recovery that our bodies talk to us, but we aren't taught to listen.

Our society says, "Eat, eat, eat… but don't look like you eat," and we are encouraged to ignore our hunger and fullness cues. We eat based on what we see and hear, not what our bodies desire internally.

But, what do our bodies want? Only they carry the truth.

In the case of PTSD, our bodies also hold our pain and trauma. The body is a brilliant work of art and it won't be ignored forever. Sooner or later, it will get our attention through aches, illness, or changes in weight.

In this way, our curves talk to us. For women who have been sexually assaulted, their bodies may gain or lose weight as a form of protection to fend off unwanted attraction and their bodies are saying: I'm here to protect you.

Perhaps my own weight loss was my body's attempt to shrink my hips and breasts and divert any male attention?

Maybe. But I knew that wasn't the kind of "protection" I needed to get better. Healing from PTSD means that we must stop hiding behind our curves or lack thereof, and face our fears head-on. Often, this requires professional help.

This is the first time I've written about my rape in a book. That's authenticity — that's curvy.

I know that I am more than what has happened to me. Getting dressed today, I felt my jeans slide over what I know to be my strong legs and hips.

I am back to me. I am back to curvy.

~Jenni Schaefer

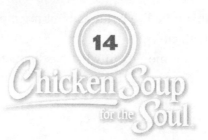

14

To Swim in the Ocean

*I have a butt, I have boobs, and I have a woman's
curves; there is no way I'd see them go to zero.*
~Jennifer Lopez, in British Elle

W hat makes a girl feel confident? Is it clothes, hair,
make-up? Maybe it's her friends?

I think it comes from within. If you are feeling
good, happy, and your life is heading in the direction
you want, then confidence emanates from your soul.

I am like many women and not a perfect size, not even close. Why
should my weight make me feel less of a person? I used to spend a lot
of time worrying about it. At times, I obsessed over it. Now, I never
think about it and I am very happy.

I have been too thin, just right, chunky and just plain "fat." I
used pants sizes to measure my worth. I believed in society's version
of "perfect" and all it did was make me feel bad about myself.

My family suffered, because if I starved I was grumpy; and if I
gained a pound, I was grumpy. It was an endless cycle of beating myself
up and never enjoying my awesome life. I had a wonderful husband
who never mentioned my weight (he said I was beautiful when I was
size 5 and when I was a size 20) and four wonderful children. But I
was too unhappy with myself to enjoy it.

Then one day everything changed: I was told I had cancer.

That's the kind of news that turns your life upside down. Being
thin wasn't as important as being alive. I had lots of time to think about

my time on earth and what I should be doing with it. I thought about my kids. My youngest was only four and she didn't deserve a grumpy mom pouting about her pants size; she deserved a mom with whom she could laugh and have crazy fun with and make great memories. So I made the choice to be happy.

When my cancer treatments were over and I felt stronger, my husband and I treated ourselves to a magical vacation. I love the ocean so my husband took me to California. I put on my swimsuit and we spent hours walking along the shore and gathering seashells and I didn't care that my suit was a size 20. I swam in the ocean and sat on the beach and held hands with my husband. I have used that swimsuit hundreds of times since then. We take the kids to the waterpark and play in the wave pool and float in the lazy river. We laugh and make memories and nobody cares what size I am.

Then one day everything changed: I was told I had cancer.

My confidence comes from within.

It's not a dress size or a bank account. It is a state of mind for which I alone am responsible. Too bad it took cancer to open my eyes.

I make sure to tell my daughters that healthy food and exercise are important, but that a size is just a size. They should be happy with themselves and swim in the ocean of life.

~Michelle Bruce

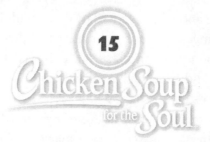

15

Through New Eyes

*Every woman that finally figured out her worth, has
picked up her suitcases of pride and boarded a flight to
freedom, which landed in the valley of change.*
~Shannon L. Alder

Struggling to pull my favorite boot-cut jeans over my
hips, I wiggled, took a deep breath and let out a sigh of
frustration. The jeans had shrunk in the dryer and they
barely fit.

"Why do I have to have such curvy hips?" I wailed, wishing for
the umpteenth time to have a slimmer shape. But that had never been
my lot in life. As soon as I started my growth spurt as a preteen, I'd
had a love-hate relationship with my hips and chest. They were too
big and unsightly and I blamed them for getting in the way while I
was playing basketball, swimming, or running.

Despite assurances from family and friends that an hourglass shape
was highly sought after, I tried unsuccessfully to alter my appearance.
Dieting, fasting, baggy clothes, double bras—I tried anything and
everything in an attempt to disguise my curves and minimize my shape.

I was a California girl, but there were no bikinis or spaghetti
straps for me. I mastered tying a sarong over my hips while lying out
at the beach. It was especially disheartening, as I had always loved
being active outdoors. Slowly, I became withdrawn and increasingly

avoided the beach.

Heading into my twenties, I got a lot of attention from the boys for my curves. I wish I could say that was a positive thing and made me appreciate my figure, but it didn't. As an introvert I hated the attention and found myself cursing my curves for a new reason. Nothing I did would alter them, despite being at a healthy weight, exercising frequently, and watching what I ate. My hips and chest were here to stay.

It wasn't until a visit with my mother in my early thirties that my relationship with my body changed. Due to a mental illness, my mother had been unable to raise me. I hadn't seen her since I was a child, and now, seeing her for the first time in twenty-two years, I realized that we had the same shape.

The exact hips and figure that I had hated with such a passion looked great on my mother.

I was mesmerized by the graceful sway of her hips as I watched her walk across the room to retrieve some photos. I realized, surprisingly, that they were the same hips and the same sway as mine. The exact hips and figure that I had hated with such a passion looked great on my mother. It was at that moment that I realized we were delightfully connected. To deny my hips was to deny my ancestry and the mom I loved.

That was the day that things changed for me. It was a long overdue turning point. I couldn't change the shape of my hips or chest, so instead, I changed the way I saw things.

I looked at my shape through new eyes. My hips were a link to my mom, and that link set me free. I started to walk taller and held my head higher with a newfound confidence, excited that I resembled my beautiful mother.

Hadn't her hips given birth to my brother and me? Hadn't my hips that so resembled hers carried me through life thus far? Through hikes, travels around the globe, down the graduation and wedding aisles and countless other places? What did it matter what size they were?

A spell was broken that day. The two aspects of my body I had disliked and tried to hide became the things I was most proud of. They were a connection to my mom, and they will carry me with confidence throughout the remainder of my life.

~Joanna Dylan

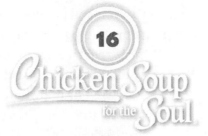

16

Baby Bump

*Giving birth and being born brings us into the essence
of creation, where the human spirit is courageous and
bold and the body, a miracle of wisdom.*
~Harriette Hartigan

Unloading my shopping cart onto the conveyer belt while juggling both children was no easy feat. The baby was perched on my hip, and the toddler was alternating between clinging to my legs and trying to escape the checkout lane. I'd already had to chase her down twice.

Time to pay. I swung the baby to my other hip so I could sign with my right hand. The toddler made another break for it while my hands were busy. A scamper of tiny shoes and she was gone again… right into the arms of a sweet, middle-aged lady who scooped her up and plopped her in my cart.

As I gathered my last bags and tried to get out of the way, I thanked this helpful lady. She just smiled and said she had been there too.

Then she placed her hand on my soft, round belly and rubbed it. "I just love baby bumps! When is this one due?"

"Well… I'm actually not pregnant. It's just left over from having two babies in less than two years."

My new friend was horrified! "I'm so sorry! I — I thought it was a baby bump… I mean, you look great! I hope I didn't embarrass you. You…"

I started laughing. "It *is* a baby bump!" I gestured to the toddler, now trying to climb out of the cart, and bounced the four-month-old a little higher on my hip. "It's my bump from that baby and this baby. It has given me my children. Why on earth would I be embarrassed about that?"

> "It's my bump from that baby and this baby. It has given me my children. Why on earth would I be embarrassed about that?"

"Well dear, just give it time. I'm sure you will lose it. You'll have your tight belly again before you know it!" And with that, she hurried out the doors, still obviously embarrassed.

Later that evening, in our oversized recliner, I was rocking the baby when the toddler crawled up onto my lap. She nuzzled her head into the soft flesh of my mama belly and let out a sigh. You could almost see the day's tension leave her little body. This is her favorite place in the whole world. Snuggled into mama's squishy middle.

So thank you, Grocery Store Lady. And yes. I love my baby bump, too.

~Jessica Ghigliotti

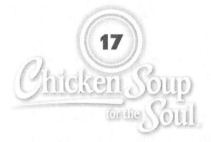

17

Picture of Health

*Enjoy yourself. These are the "good old days" you're
going to miss in the years ahead.*
~Author Unknown

"One, two, three, smile," my husband Lonny said. My oldest son, the first of five boys, put his arm around me and we grinned. It was the end of summer and he was heading back to graduate school. An internship had kept him close to home for one last season, and the picture together was the finale of the many sweet family times we'd had over the past three months.

"Want to look at these?" Lonny asked. He handed me my iPhone. I looked through the photos and smiled at the images of my son. Handsome. Strong. But my pictures? My arms were thicker than usual, and there was a gentle swell to my tummy. I'd always worked very hard, depriving myself often, to stay on the slim side. Now I was about 10 pounds heavier than usual. I made a mental note to work on it.

"This one will be great," I said, handing the phone to my son.

"It's nice!" he said.

"It's perfect," Lonny said.

In the picture, our smiles came from the heart as the setting sun stretched behind us. It was a sweet shot and I was excited to post it on Facebook.

Just as soon as I cropped it.

I'd be humiliated to share the shot as it was—weeks of carelessness, thick and evident on my body. When my waistline changed, so did my self-value and esteem.

I'm a tall lady, just over six feet. If I'm asked to be exact, I say I'm 5'13". Many people, when they comment on my height, add that it must be nice. The height must enable me to gain weight without noticing. I haven't found that to be true. After delivering a couple of my boys, I carried extra weight for quite a few months. It always came off with just a bit of effort. But recently, it was harder to maintain the weight that I wanted. I liked to be low on the BMI chart. I felt good when people complimented me on being slender after having so many kids. It filled me up — even if my tummy was sometimes empty.

> *When my waistline changed, so did my self-value and esteem.*

Hormones and mid-life body changes had altered my ability to live as a lightweight, though. Keeping that weight meant more deprivation and more runs in the mornings. And because I love to cook and bake and gather my men around the dining room table, it meant a struggle.

Over the next few days the entire family participated in preparations before our son's return to school, helping him pack and loading boxes into his car. And I planned one last family dinner. Bringing the family together, sharing food and talk was everything to me. It would be a long time before it would happen again.

"What would you like to eat for your last dinner home?" I asked my son.

"Homemade pizza," he said.

Years ago, I fell in love with making my own pizza crust. Just a drop of honey gave it a gentle touch of sweet. And I'd just about replicated the sauce and seasonings on the pizza at our favorite restaurant.

Later that night, we strung up lights on the patio and played our favorite 1940's music as I served the pizza and savored the sound of my united family sharing stories and laughter.

"How about you, Shawnelle?" Lonny asked, noticing that my plate had only salad. "No pizza for you?"

I shook my head. But my family ate heartily and they were on second slices when Lonny took out his phone.

"Boys, lean in," he said. "Let me get a picture of you with your mom."

The boys gathered around me and my youngest wrapped his arms around my neck. We smiled and laughed as Lonny took a few shots. When I looked at the photo, it spoke to my heart. The strong bond we shared was evident in the joy in our smiles.

And suddenly, it didn't matter that I wasn't as thin as I'd been before.

The changes in my body were the result of togetherness with the people I love the most. We'd shared good times and the result was good. The curve of my tummy shouldn't bother me — after all, I grew five sons right there, under the beat of my very own heart.

"Hey, Mom," my son said. "There's a slice of pizza left. I think it belongs to you."

He served me and I smiled. I looked around the table and was deeply grateful for every moment of summer family time, and for this last night together.

I was a curvier version of what I'd been summers before, but life was beautiful. And I was, too.

The pictures showed it all.

I was healthy and content.

~Shawnelle Eliasen

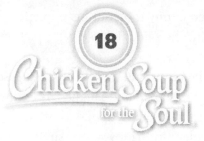

18

Cankles

To be fully seen by somebody, then, and be
loved anyhow — this is a human offering
that can border on miraculous.
~Elizabeth Gilbert, Committed: A Skeptic
Makes Peace with Marriage

"I hate my legs," my wife said.

"I love your legs," I said. "What's wrong with them?"

"Instead of thin, sexy ankles, I've got cankles."

"What in the world are cankles?"

"My ankles are so thick that my calves go straight down into my feet. I don't have ankles, I've got cankles; calves and feet, but no ankles."

I first saw Neecey more than two decades ago at a bar in Pittsburgh. A large group of runners, all members of People Who Run Downtown, had gathered to run and then have a meal. I noticed a foxy lady sitting with a couple of runners I knew. She had curly blond hair that framed her cute, petite face like a fashion photo.

The following week, a mutual runner friend introduced us before the run and after a bit of small talk, I mentioned I was a jazz and blues musician and asked Neecey if she liked blues music.

"I love the blues! It's my favorite genre of music."

I invited her to a concert that Saturday night, a few days later, in which some friends would be performing and she eagerly accepted and gave me her phone number. But when I called her the next day, and several times after that, I got a "phone not in service" message. She must have been too shy to say no to the date and gave me a phony number, I thought.

The following week when I saw her at the running group, I asked her about the wrong number.

"Oh my God! I can't believe I did that. I was so nervous when you asked me out that I gave you the first six digits of my work number and the last four of my home number. Meanwhile, I was feeling really bad because you didn't call. I thought you didn't want to go out with me."

To make a long story short, she gave me the correct number and we were married a year later.

In 2004 we were both devastated to learn that Neecey had breast cancer. The doctor told us she would need surgery and radiation but chances for a cure were good. That night we snuggled on the couch, both teary eyed.

> *"During the course of our marriage, my love for you has gone much deeper than your physical charms, great as they are."*

"There is something we need to talk about," she said. "The doctor said the surgery would leave me with a misshapen breast. He offered reconstructive surgery if I want it. I'll have it if you think I should, so I won't look like a freak to you when I'm naked. But you know how much I fear doctors, hospitals, and especially surgery."

I took Neecey's hand in mind. "Babe, I fell in love with you and everything that makes you what you are: your soul, your spirit, your personality and your pouty way when we disagree. During the course of our marriage, my love for you has gone much deeper than your physical charms, great as they are. The important thing is to get rid of cancer. I want your body to be your body after surgery, not a remade, fabricated thing the doctors have put together. I want the woman I married, not some reconstruction project."

The surgery and radiation were a success and five years later, Neecey was declared cancer free. She has a small incision below the nipple that, with the loss of tissue, makes the breast point downward. It has the odd but cute look of a closed eye.

This brings us back to my conversation two weeks ago with Neecey about her cankles.

"Babe, in case you've forgotten, you have a picture perfect runner's body and a face I'd fight the Mongolian horde for. I'm more than willing to accept your cankles in the bargain."

~Ray Budd

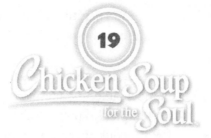

19

An Art Perspective

*When you judge a woman by her appearance, it
doesn't define her. It defines you.*
~Dr. Steve Maraboli

I have been involved in the art world all my life, as a student, creator and consumer. Early in my studies I became aware of a dramatic change in the body shape of the typical female subject.

Paintings created before the First World War showed healthy, full-figured women. The change in body type seems to have happened during the "flapper" craze that swept across Europe and North America. The female shape depicted in paintings moved away from the traditional, fuller figure — perhaps reflecting the deprivations brought about by two world wars, when food was scarce and malnutrition common. But even though conditions improved, the female shape in art did not revert back. And today, we are bombarded with depictions of skinny bodies in art that would have been unacceptable before the turn of the century.

The origin of the curvy female form in art is lost in the mists of time. The earliest examples of cave drawing and sculpture found in Europe and the Americas depict the rounded, full-figured, well-fed female form. These early artists would never have considered representing any other shape to depict a female. The ideal bodies preferred by master painters like Renoir, Rubens and Matisse were what we now define as plus-sized women. Peter Paul Rubens, the famous classicist painter, even lent his name to the painting of robust healthy women. A perfect female sitter was given the complimentary description of being "Rubenesque."

Early in my art history studies I took a class in life drawing. Each week a new professional model sat for us, alternating between male and female sitters. The tutor attempted to provide a variety of body types, but in spite of her best efforts, all of the art models looked similar: They were slim if female, and thin and muscular if male.

Halfway through the term the teacher announced that she had secured the services of her favorite model, Elizabeth. She had been one of our tutor's private sitters but had never sat for a class of students. Elizabeth was very shy and knew we usually used models on the skinny side, which she was not, so she was uncertain of the reception she might receive. Still, our teacher convinced her to give it a try.

We were told that having Elizabeth pose would be such a treat we had better not miss out on the opportunity.

"What makes Elizabeth so special?" I asked the teacher.

In my naiveté, I thought that the main demand on a model was being able to sit still for an hour or so.

"Wait and see," said the teacher. "It will be a revelation, I promise."

The following week Elizabeth arrived. All of the students were surprised when she took her place in front of the class. Elizabeth was a large, middle-aged woman, much different from any of the other life drawing models. Some of the female students looked slightly askance at our new visitor. They obviously had other expectations. There were some furtively exchanged glances and even some giggles.

Elizabeth quickly settled down to the task at hand. It was wonderful to see how every movement of her body, or of the drapery she wore, changed the light and shade on her wonderful shape. She exuded a feeling of comfort, warmth and a pride in her full figure, and sensed what the group needed — happily responding to requests for a change in pose. Elizabeth had a great sense of self and this came across in her confident and creative manner and then manifested itself in our work.

As predicted by our teacher, she turned out to be the highlight of the year.

Before the end of the class everyone was asking when our new favourite model would be back. Elizabeth was delighted at our enthusiasm and volunteered to return and sit for us for the rest of the semester. All the girls in the class, looking suitably sheepish, lined up to hug Elizabeth as she was getting ready to leave. Wrapped up in those hugs and smiles were silent apologies for being quick to judge.

> *The classical painters had it right when it came to understanding the ideal shape of a woman.*

We never used thin models again during that course. The classical painters had it right when it came to understanding the ideal shape of a woman. It's up to us to help redefine it for future generations.

~James A. Gemmell

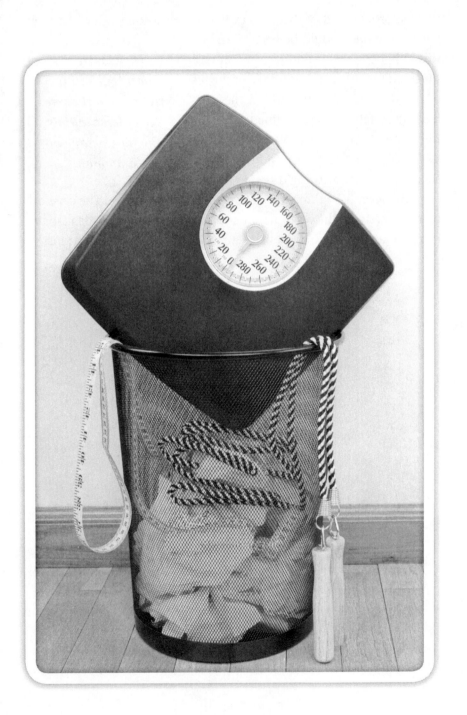

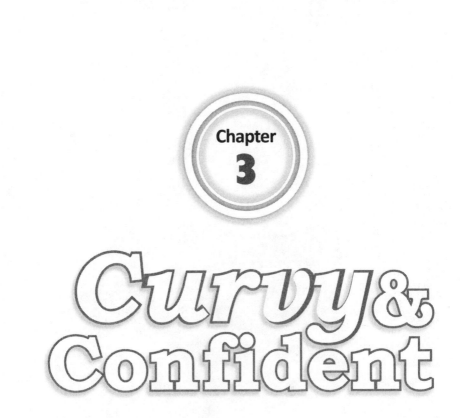

Chapter
3

Curvy &
Confident

Sharing the Wisdom

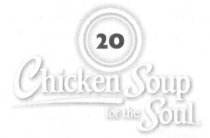

Bad Mama Jama

*I think that whatever size or shape body you have, it's
important to embrace it and get down!*
~Christina Aguilera, Marie Claire

While I was working as a tutor at Piedmont Technical College in Greenwood, South Carolina, I worked with a student named Darla. When I first met her, she couldn't look me in the eye while talking to me. She also had problems with anxiety and got so nervous around people that she literally shook. Basically, she was a mess.

As I tutored Darla in math, she began to open up and share her background. She had previously been a swimsuit model and had won swimsuit competitions run by some mainstream companies. In fact, she met her ex-husband at one of these competitions. At the beginning of their marriage, she said, she had been like a trophy for him and he loved showing her off to other men. As their marriage progressed, he became more and more controlling. A few years into their marriage, Darla got pregnant. After giving birth, she had trouble losing weight. This angered her husband and he became even more abusive. After years of his abuse, Darla left.

By the time I met her, Darla's self-esteem was shot. Prior to her marriage, she equated her value to her looks. Now weighing more than she ever had before, and having been abused and belittled for years by her husband, she thought she only had value as a mother.

She shared that she was attracted to a gentleman we both knew.

Unfortunately, she was sure that because he was so attractive and she had gained weight, there was no way he would be interested in her.

The curious thing was that Darla saw beauty in me. She said she wished she looked like me. Now, I am way bigger than Darla. We aren't even close in size. I'm not an average plus-size woman; I'm super-plus and I've got hips and thighs for days. And even though she didn't know it, the guy she liked was hitting on me daily. So I knew it wasn't about looks. It was all about Darla's confidence.

One day, as we walked into the Teaching and Learning Center for a tutoring session, Darla commented that when we entered the room, every man turned and watched me. I knew this was my chance to show her something that would begin to shift her thinking.

I asked Darla, "How did I walk into this room? Did I walk in like I owned the building? Did I walk in with my head up and shoulders back like I was the baddest thing moving, like I heard "She's A Bad Mama Jama" playing just for me? Or did I walk in with my head down like I was afraid or ashamed of who I was?"

"You walked in with confidence," Darla said.

I asked her if I was the size of a model, or if I was one of the larger women in the room.

"You are a larger woman," she said, "but it didn't seem to matter. You are beautiful and everybody knew it."

Then I told her something that I would repeat to her many times in the coming months and something that I have shared with many women since then. "The thing that will always command attention is confidence," I said. "I walked in here like I was the baddest thing moving, and in their minds they wanna know what I know that makes me walk with such confidence. A real man is looking for a real woman, a whole woman. He's not looking for some broken down woman that he has to piece together. A real man, a King, is looking for a Queen who can rule and reign with him. A real man is looking for a real woman who knows who she is and loves herself."

I know Darla didn't believe me, but she smiled and nodded. Every time we met to go over her math, I would take the opportunity to build her up and tell her how awesome she was. That semester ended and I continued to tutor her in another math class, making sure to speak life into her every chance I got. I often wondered if my words were sinking in.

Time went on and Darla graduated and I thought I would never see her again. Then one day, about six months after graduation, Darla came to campus for career counseling and came looking for me.

I couldn't believe my eyes. The woman who couldn't look me in the eye when we first met, who trembled from nervousness and never smiled, was now smiling from ear to ear. She looked amazing!

The Darla I knew rarely took time with her appearance because she felt like her weight made her unattractive, so why try? Now she had her hair and make-up done and was wearing the cutest outfit.

But that smile told the real tale.

Darla ran and hugged me. She thanked

> *"The thing that will always command attention is confidence," I said. "I walked in here like I was the baddest thing moving."*

me for everything I said and did for her. She told me that it took some time, but one day it clicked; she realized she was worthy of living an awesome life and she decided to do just that. She told me that she would never forget what I had done for her and that she was making a deliberate effort to make the same type of impact in her daughters' lives.

Also, she'd gotten up the courage to approach our mutual friend and was waiting to see if he would make the move to call her. And then she said the best thing of all.

"I hope he calls, but if he doesn't, I'll be fine. That just means there's someone else out there who will appreciate me for who I am. If he doesn't call, it will be his loss."

"Girl, you are so right," I said. "And you know why?"

Without missing a beat, she said: "Yes! 'Cause I'm a Bad Mama Jama!"

~Regina Sunshine Robinson

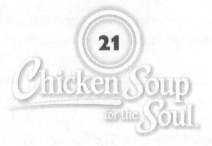

I Am Woman

Self-trust is the first secret of success.
~Ralph Waldo Emerson

I'm standing at the front of a conference room filled with 100 mompreneurs, hard working women who just spent the day learning how to grow their businesses while juggling their family lives. It's my turn on stage and I have eight minutes to get my message of radical self-love through to them.

I've picked the song "Woman (Oh Mama)" by Joy Williams to play, and I ask everyone to kick off their heels and get ready to dance with me. As the song begins, I take a deep breath and start the talk I have been practicing.

"I'd like you to place your hands on your belly and take a few deep breaths. Ninety-one percent of women have an I-hate-my-body moment every day, and our poor bellies get the brunt of that, especially for those of us who have been through childbirth. So let's send some love to the belly."

I hear a few giggles of recognition in the audience, and I know they are with me. I lead the women through some dance moves: Hip circles, symbolic of childbirth, represent the businesses they are birthing; Breast circles represent nourishing their businesses. This one gets a lot of laughs. I love looking out and seeing that they are having fun and not judging how they look. This is what I want for them to remember, that their bodies can be a source of joy.

"As women, we are constantly told to make ourselves small. But you have big dreams you want to grow, so you need to know that you have a right to take up space in this world. Take up space now, stretch your arms out and give your dreams wings to fly!" The room is full of waving arms and smiling faces, a beautiful sight.

The song is nearing the finish, and I ask the women to repeat after me: "I. AM. WOMAN."

A joyful chorus of raised voices ends the song. It's time for me to bring the message home.

"And now, I'd like you to take a minute to place your hands on your bellies again and close your eyes. Imagine you are getting ready for your day and you look in the mirror. What is the first thought that comes to your mind?"

> *But you have big dreams you want to grow, so you need to know that you have a right to take up space in this world.*

"Ugh!" says a woman in the front of the room.

"Ugh? This is what I hear from many women," I say. "But I want you to think about how you are putting that negativity onto yourself energetically, then going out into the world to promote your business, which is *you*.

"Instead, when you are getting ready in the morning and you look in the mirror, I want you to send love to the woman you see. Because she is worthy, she is beautiful, and she has big dreams. You need to give her love so she can go out and do her great work in this world."

My time on stage is done, and I step down hoping that my words hit home. I hope that these one hundred women remember this moment the next day, as they are getting ready for work. Body love does not happen overnight, but the first step is paying attention to when those "ugh" moments happen. Often they have become so much a part of our daily routine, we don't realize we are doing it to ourselves.

There is a line in "Woman (Oh Mama)" that keeps running through my head: "I am the universe wrapped in skin."

I love the expansiveness of this image, how each of us contains beautiful multitudes and limitless possibilities inside our skin.

My wish is for every woman to embrace herself for the universe inside of her.

~Joyelle Brandt

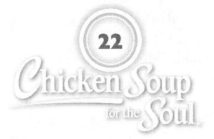

22

Comfortable in My Shorts

*A smile is the light in the window of your face that
tells people you're at home.*
~Author Unknown

I had been going through a period of negative self-talk, wondering how other people viewed me. Did they just see a "fat" woman? Were they able to see a person, or were they judging me by my size?

And then one day, I literally bumped into someone who changed my life. I was at the grocery store, after having spent thirty minutes at home trying to find something to wear that was cute and didn't make me feel fat. I was so frazzled by the time I left for the store that I had forgotten my list, and I was pushing my cart through the canned vegetables aisle trying to remember what I needed. That's when I ran into the lady.

As I was apologizing, I stopped mid-sentence, because she simply shook her head, with her hand toward me as if to say "no apology necessary." I saw how happy and positive she was. Her smile seemed confident, friendly and encouraging. It showed wisdom and grace, while her eyes showed strength and kindness.

After we untangled our carts and walked away, I found myself thinking, *Wow, I wish I could be like her.* That's when a quiet thought came to me. *What is it about her that you want to have? Her smile, her kindness, or her body and weight?* I came to a complete stop as I realized something. I had no idea how big or small she was. I hadn't noticed if she was thin or plump. I didn't see her size. What I cared about was her smile, because that was how she showed she cared.

After that, I started looking at people a new way, evaluating whether I was noticing their looks or their attitudes. I realized that I was not noticing their size — no, I was seeing their other attributes. If they smiled and we made a connection, I didn't look past that and consider their weight.

> *I didn't see her size. What I cared about was her smile, because that was how she showed she cared.*

That was the lesson I took away from this encounter, what I carry with me all the time now — people will remember my smile and my kindness more than my size. I also realized that it was my own thoughts and words that led people to focus on my weight.

If I acted like I couldn't do things with them because I didn't want to be seen in a swimsuit or shorts, then guess what they would think about? But if I talked about my accomplishments, my passions and goals, they would follow my lead,

Now, I'm walking with confidence again, believing I can put my best foot forward and it will be enough. I can make a difference, show kindness and love, change the world… and I can do that wearing a size 0 or a size 16. Because it's not about size. It's about attitude and how you treat people.

I'm comfortable in my shorts, spider veins and all. I am more than a size, and I am so excited to see where this new attitude will lead me.

~Lydia Young-Samson

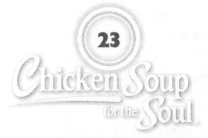

23

A Flowering

An angel can illuminate the thought and mind of man
by strengthening the power of vision.
~St. Thomas Aquinas

I grew up during a time when shopping for what we now call "plus-size clothing" was torture. I had to go to the "misses" or teen department even though I was only eight years old.

I was always the youngest person shopping in the stores that carried clothing my mom felt was appropriate for me. The clothes were more middle-aged church lady than high school student. Feeling I had no choice, I accepted that those were indeed the clothes for me.

Eventually, I came to believe that "invisible" was the way I should dress. I shouldn't seek out clothing that hugged my curves; instead, I should seek to have a big swath of black cloth swallow me up.

This was how I bought my clothes until I was in my twenties. And then, a few years ago, I was exchanging an ill-fitting swath of dark cloth I had bought a week earlier for a wedding. When I presented the outfit to the young saleslady at the cash register, she looked confused.

"Are these clothes for you?" she asked.

I was completely flustered. Why was she asking me this?

"Um... yes," I admitted.

"No way," she said, shaking her head. "I am not selling these clothes to you. You are too young for these!"

I was in shock, but before I could protest, she came around the counter, took me by the hand, and showed me several beautiful pieces that had color, patterns and shape. She showed me clothes that I always figured were not for me — I had been told as much, and unfortunately, had believed it.

Before I left the store, my sales angel gave me some advice: "Those clothes you were planning to buy — don't buy clothes like that ever again. Don't hide yourself."

I nodded and smiled. For the rest of the day, I couldn't stop thinking about her advice. An amazing thing had happened. A seed was planted, not only in my mind but also in my heart. Something in me had shifted when I bought a coral-colored blouse for the wedding! It was a life affirming purchase. It's pretty difficult to hide while wearing coral.

> *"Don't buy clothes like that ever again. Don't hide yourself."*

Each time I bought clothes after that crucial day, I looked for items I liked, not items that someone else might think were acceptable for my body. I chose colors that complemented my skin tone and made my heart smile. I bought clothes in my actual size — not ones that would swallow me up and hide me!

Each of those decisions watered the seeds planted that day, and gradually, I began to bloom.

There have been a few times in my life when someone has encouraged and guided me. These encounters have ultimately led to new ways of thinking and living for me. I remember how significant and empowered I felt that someone took the time to assure and mentor me, simply because they cared. Girls need to know that no matter their size they are important, and so are their ideas and choices. They need to know that their worth has nothing to do with their dress size and we are all valid and valuable.

That is what I felt that day the saleslady refused to sell me an outfit. I didn't know it then, but it was one of the best things that could have ever happened to me.

A few years ago I saw my sales angel again. I told her how she had changed my life. I was able to thank her and encourage her to continue planting those beneficial seeds, because once they take root and blossom, the fruit produced is shared with others, so they too can blossom.

~Maxine Young

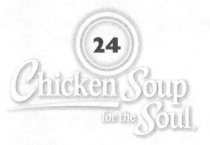

Just the Way You Are

Be bold and love your body. STOP FIXING IT.
It was never broken.
~Eve Ensler, The Good Body

I had just placed an armload of magazines in the "free" box when two teenage girls entered the library's foyer. They brushed snow off their heads and stomped their boots on the heavy mat and jostled one another playfully.

While one of the girls made a phone call, her friend, a slightly "curvier" blonde, wandered over and dug through the magazines I had just put down. Combing through the books in the box beside her, I watched her flip through the slick pages.

I have battled my weight since I was a kid. Because of that I've been an avid reader of health and fitness magazines, hoping to find the secret to weight maintenance. I used to read these magazines cover to cover, feeling like every article told me another thing that was wrong with my body.

It's taken time and hard work to remind myself of my worth. Now, I read these magazines for suggestions and helpful tips, not because I think they will "fix" me. My family tends to run large, and so do I. I work out and eat decently most of the time. Sometimes I eat cookies. I'm not broken.

As the girl's friend chattered in the background, the one beside me stopped on a page. I glanced over. The photos were familiar. I knew it was an article about losing weight. That magazine seems to have one every week. This one was drastic, recommending you eat a boatload of cabbage soup and not much else. I remember the story had made me so angry, I nearly wrote a letter to the editor.

Once upon a time, I would have rushed out and loaded my cart with all of the ingredients for that soup. I had even been tempted to go on the diet for a friend's upcoming wedding. I hadn't seen my friend in nearly a year and I'd gained some weight and was self-conscious about the extra pounds.

> *I used to read these magazines cover to cover, feeling like every article told me another thing that was wrong with my body.*

Instead, next to the article, I had angrily written a counter message to myself in the margin: *"You are beautiful just the way you are."*

My face flushed as the girl read my angry scribbles. I felt like my private thoughts were on display. I hoped she hadn't noticed I was the one who dropped the magazines in the box.

"Ready?" Miss Formerly on the Phone asked.

"Go ahead. I'm going to go to the bathroom first," said the girl, holding the magazine.

As her friend shrugged and left the foyer to enter the main library, I feverishly dug through the books to hide my embarrassment. Surely this girl wasn't going to ask me about what I had written? As much as this seemed like my cue to leave too, I couldn't. What was she going to do?

I heard a ripping sound and turned involuntarily. The girl smiled and looked away as she tucked a page she had removed into her jacket pocket without a word. Then she walked away.

For all I knew she was going to pull out the article and laugh about it with her friend. But somehow, I didn't think so. Maybe this girl would look at my scribble in the margin and grow up not dieting, not reading silly articles that made her feel flawed.

Maybe she would grow up knowing she is beautiful just the way she is.

~Drema Sizemore Drudge

Sharing the Wisdom | 83

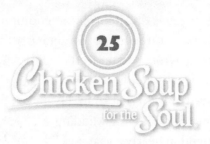

Missing Body Parts

Be present in all things and thankful for all things.
~Maya Angelou

While rummaging through a drawer in search of an old photograph, I came across a picture of a teenage girl. Dressed in a navy and gold pep club uniform, she'd positioned her pompoms to cover each hip. Her blond hair cascaded past her shoulders. My eyes followed the blondness downward and then stopped abruptly — someone had snipped her legs off with a pair of scissors.

I tossed the photo aside and continued my search.

I found more photos of this girl, from her teen years through to motherhood. In one picture she resembled a skeleton, with her gaunt frame and protruding cheekbones; in another, she looked three times bigger. I found plenty of in-between ones, too. These photos, too, had missing body parts — whole legs, thighs, her derrière, even an upper arm had vanished.

My heart ached for this young woman. What had made her despise her body so much that she had cut it up and thrown away pieces of it? I wished I could travel back in time to speak with her.

If I could talk to that long-ago girl, I'd encourage her to cherish, nourish, strengthen, and care for her body. This magnificent creation of flesh and blood hopefully has a long road ahead and will carry her through a lifetime. Thanks to her body, she can feel, see, hear, walk, touch, and maybe even bear children one day. With it, she can hold her loved ones close, feel the warmth of the sunshine, or wipe away a teardrop.

I'd remind her that many of the greatest, most celebrated, successful women throughout history were curvy, confident, and beautiful. And that all the dieting in the world won't make her happy — it will just cost her money, time, health, and her sanity.

I'd encourage her to discover her strengths, talents, and pursue her dreams.

These photos, too, had missing body parts.

I'd remind her that size should never define who or what she is. The size of her waist, hips, or thighs is not nearly as great as the size of her heart.

I'd tell her that life is too short to wear only black, and that she should wear what makes her feel alive and beautiful.

And I'd tell her that everyone deserves to be pampered and spoiled. So she should soak in a candlelight bath, eat that ice cream cone, and savor that glass of wine.

Because one day, she'll look back on those old photographs and wish she had lived, laughed, and loved more. But thankfully, it's never too late to change your attitude and love yourself.

I know... because I'm the one in the photographs, the girl with the missing body parts. And now I'm whole.

~Jill Burns

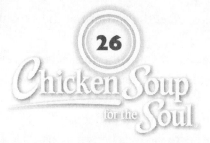

The Curvy Sister

To be beautiful means to be yourself. You don't need to
be accepted by others. You need to accept yourself.
~Thich Nhat Hanh

I was born the third of nine children, but growing up, people always assumed I was the oldest. I was taller than one older sister and more filled out than the other. It was a source of pride for me in some regards. I could hit a softball farther, run faster, and raid Mom's closet at an earlier age. My size threw our family pecking order out the window, as my older sisters viewed me as their equal instead of a pesky little sister. I felt more than just confident about the way I looked; I felt unique and special, and I never gave my size or shape much thought. I was just happy to be me.

That changed one fall afternoon when I was thirteen. I was hanging out with one of my best friends, a boy my age who had yet to hit his growth spurt. He was shorter than me, pencil thin, and really funny. We hung out whenever we could and talked about everything under the sun. Maybe that's why he thought it was okay to say something that changed how I saw myself for years to come.

We sat in my back yard, under the shade of a massive oak tree. It was one of those completely ordinary afternoons. I found a small stick in the grass and slowly peeled the bark away with my fingernail while we talked about things like school and homework. Then I glanced up to find him looking at me with a rather cryptic smile on his face. I knew this expression all too well — it usually meant he had something he really wanted to tell me. I expected he had a juicy bit of gossip to share, or maybe one of his funny stories, but I never expected what actually came out of his mouth.

"You won't believe what my mom said last night," he said, watching me out of the corner of his eye. I didn't find this strange at first. He was always fighting with his mom about something. But then he said, "Oh, no. Never mind. I can't tell you."

Something in his voice got my attention. I suddenly had the feeling that whatever his mom said was about me. I wasn't particularly worried though, because she and I had always liked each other. I sat up a little straighter and looked at him. "Oh, come on," I said. "You can't say something like that and then not tell me."

He squirmed uncomfortably and shook his head. "No, I can't tell you." A nervous shiver ran through me. I had the sense that maybe she said something not-so-nice about me. But there was no going back now. I had to know.

"Oh, come on." I punched his shoulder. "Just tell me."

"Okay. She said…" he paused for a dramatic, deep breath. "She said you have a chunky butt and chunky legs."

For a moment or two, I just sat there, staring stupidly at the nervous smile on his face. A thousand thoughts raced through my mind: *How could she say that? Did she, someone I had always trusted, really think that or was he making this up? Why would he say something like this to me? Did he think it was funny? Did he think it was true?* And worst of all: *Was she right? Was there something wrong with the way my body looked?*

I imagine my face went white, then red. My throat felt tight with tears, but I refused to cry in front of him. By the time I staggered to my feet and began speed walking to the back door, my friend knew he had made a terrible mistake. He hurried to catch up. "Wait! Where are you going?" he asked.

I shoved him away and said, "I'm going inside."

He jumped in front of me and said, "Are you mad?"

Was I mad? Obviously. "What is wrong with you?" I finally yelled.

"Why would you say that to me?"

I ran into my house, slammed the door, and hurried to my room. I barely made it there before the tears came. I no longer felt unique and special, or proud to be me. I felt ugly and broken.

Later that night, in a rare display of teenage wisdom, I opened up to my parents about what happened. When I got to the "chunky butt and chunky legs" part, I wanted to curl up and disappear. I could barely get the words past my lips. But I forced them out, unable to look at my parents as I finished recounting what happened. I stared at the brown living room carpet instead, holding my breath and waiting for one of two things. Either they would tell me she was right or they would become indignant and angry and tell me she was wrong.

> *In a world of impossible ideals and a thousand different definitions for what makes a person attractive, there is only one opinion that really matters. Mine.*

But my dad did neither. He simply said, "What do you think? Do you think she's right?"

This surprised me, but I mulled it over. My jeans were a size 6. No matter how I felt about my body, I couldn't call a size 6 "fat." I said to Dad, "No. I don't think she's right."

Dad sat back. "Then that's all that matters."

I left the room not quite convinced that Dad was right about this. It seemed too simple a solution. For many years to come, that afternoon stuck with me. As much as I wanted to be happy with my body, I couldn't fully take Dad's advice. Instead, I tried to make peace through diets, exercise, and creative clothing choices.

It's taken me nearly thirty years to realize Dad knew what he was talking about after all.

I am now twice the size I was that day, but I'm happy to be me again. I see my curves as a sign that I'm healthy and strong, and I wouldn't want to be anyone else. And I've learned a valuable lesson along the way: In a world of impossible ideals and a thousand different definitions for what makes a person attractive, there is only one

opinion that really matters. Mine.
And I think I am beautiful.

~Debra Mayhew

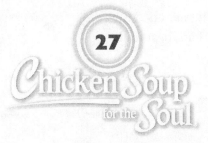

27

The Lesson

Talk to yourself like you would to someone you love.
~Brené Brown

I tried on the dress and looked at myself. My first thought was, *This dress looks amazing.* Then I inspected myself closely, looking at all my stretch marks. The dress looked amazing, but on me, it was hideous. I sat down and looked at myself in the mirror, my self-confidence shattered.

"You okay? My elder sister knocked from the other side of the changing room door. "What's taking so long?"

"Coming, Jiji!" I said.

I dressed back up into my clothes and went outside.

"Didn't you try on the dress? Why did you change?" she asked.

"Jiji, don't you think I am a little plump for these dresses." I stated it more like a fact than asking it.

"Come with me," Jiji said, tugging me, and she led me to the Pizza Hut.

"We will have a double cheese pizza with two truffle pastries, thanks," my sister told the waiter. "Those are your favourites, right?" she asked me.

"Yes Jiji, but…"

"But?"

"Jiji, I am fat."

"So?"

"Umm…"

"Look at that man there," my sister said. "What are you thinking about him?"

"Nothing."

"Okay, now look around you. Are you thinking anything about anyone else here?"

"No."

"But you are thinking about yourself. Right?"

"Yes."

"And don't you think you are giving too much importance to what others might think of you?"

I couldn't say anything. I just looked down.

"I am saying this to make you understand that you must learn to love yourself," she said. "Your opinion about you matters; nobody else's opinion matters."

> *I needed to accept my curves and more than that—own them, and be proud of myself.*

I smiled and said nothing. She was right, I needed to love myself. I needed to accept my curves and more than that—own them, and be proud of myself.

Midway through our lunch, I had a thought: "Jiji, I liked that dress. It looked amazing on me. Can we go and buy it?"

"Sure," my sister smiled. "I am proud of you."

I was proud of myself, too. My curves and stretch marks are a part of my identity. Now when I have weak moments, I look at the dress Jiji bought for me and I smile, remembering my sister's lesson.

~Mudita Raj

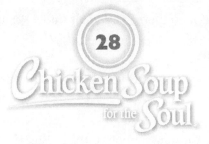

28

The Truth

*I was always looking outside myself for strength
and confidence but it comes from within.
It is there all the time.*
~Anna Freud

I was in my forties before I learned the truth about my mother… and the truth about myself. My sister had put together a montage of photos in celebration of my parents' wedding anniversary. I watched as images depicting forty years of life and love flashed across my computer screen: my mother beaming at the camera as a nineteen-year-old bride; mom cradling my newborn sister in her arms.

As each photo documenting every momentous occasion of Mom and Dad's life together appeared, I was surprised by what I saw. The pictures of Mom showed a very different version of the person I remembered from my childhood. She'd been overweight my entire life (her words, not mine) but the woman in the slideshow was anything but big. She was curvier in some seasons of life than others, but absolutely beautiful, with a body most women would love to have.

This could only mean one thing: All those years Mom told us how big she was, all of those ridiculous fad diets she tried and the Jazzercise classes I was dragged to… were all for a big "fat" lie. A lie I believed because Mom said it was true. The truly sad thing is… I'm sure Mom believed it, too.

I jumped up from my computer and headed for the closet. I

climbed up a stepladder and carefully removed a box containing two decades of my own family memories. I carried it to my bed and opened the lid, uncertain of what I might find.

Like Mom, I struggled with body image as a young woman and spent a small fortune on exercise tapes, weight-loss pills, and gimmicky diets. Health had never been a motivating factor; it had always been about changing my appearance. I wanted to be skinny. Besides the five minutes I spent as a size 6 in the late 1990's, I'd always thought of myself as grossly overweight. But the pictures I now thumbed through told a different story. The truth is, I hadn't been fat at all! I was holding the proof in my hands.

> *But the pictures I now thumbed through told a different story. The truth is, I hadn't been fat at all!*

I shook my head. My son and daughter had grown up hearing me speak the same self-deprecating lies about my weight that my mother had told herself. I could only hope they hadn't grown up believing them. I cringed at the thought.

Oh, how I wished I could go back in time! I would have told my mom how beautiful she was. I would have spent less time criticizing my own appearance and more time teaching my children the importance of loving yourself from the inside out. Positive self-image — being confident in every perfectly imperfect part of one's body — it really does start at home. Women have diverse shapes and whether they are a size 2 or 22, we are all "real" women, each one of us beautiful in our own way.

This is the truth I hope my own children will know — a truth that took me far too long to learn.

~Melissa Wootan

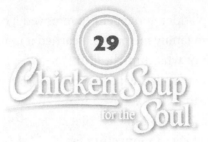

29

A Beautiful Reflection

To love is nothing. To be loved is something. But to
love and be loved, that's everything.
~T. Tolis

very day I would look in the mirror, hate what I saw, but repeat the words, "I am beautiful." I didn't do it willingly. Sometimes I'd cry or grit my teeth to get the words out. But I kept saying it, no matter what.

It was at the request of my boyfriend that I began the daily ritual. He was drawn to me because of my kindness, gentle spirit and love of silliness. But, he also saw me as beautiful and it bothered him that I couldn't see it myself.

For a long time I had accepted the lie that my weight made me a second-rate person undeserving of romance, popularity or success. Years of rejection and being ignored had caused me to build a cocoon around myself. I mistakenly thought that if I stayed quiet, maybe I would be safe. Lonely, but safe.

I wrapped myself in layers of fears and phobias, my heart breaking a little more with each wedding invitation or engagement announcement. I gave up hoping for my true love, convinced I wasn't good enough.

It wasn't until I resolved to be happy on my own that I met him and things began to change. He pointed out my positive qualities, best features and most admirable character traits, making me repeat them out loud. It felt awkward. I was embarrassed. I laughed, and I cried. But, I kept at it every day: "I am beautiful."

And then, one day, an amazing thing happened. Staring in the mirror, I realized with a shock that I believed it! He wasn't lying or just being nice. It was true! I am beautiful!

The layers of my cocoon slowly dissolved, and as I left behind the security of aloneness, new wings unfurled in vibrant colors and I learned to fly.

Today, the boyfriend who changed my life and taught me to love myself is my husband of fourteen years. He still loves my curves and has taught me to be confident

For a long time I had accepted the lie that my weight made me a second-rate person undeserving of romance, popularity or success.

and proud no matter what my dress size. He encourages me to be as healthy and fit as possible, but I know now that my beauty encompasses every part of who I am.

I am caring. I am talented. I am worthy. I am beautiful.

~L. Joy Douglas

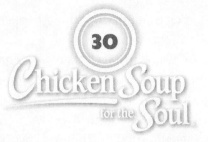

30

Letter to My Twelve-Year-Old Self

Knowledge is a process of piling up facts; wisdom
lies in their simplification.
~Martin H. Fischer

Old letters are like time capsules. They are precious and illuminating, but they can also be bittersweet. It's endearing to see ourselves at a younger age, but it's also frustrating not to be able to give our young selves advice that could save us heartache later on. Recently, my cousin Nena sent me back a letter I'd written to her almost forty years ago, when I was twelve.

Here it is, word for word:

March 23, 1977

Dear Nena,

Today is my mom's birthday and Bobby, me, and Stevie got her a big, fancy carving knife and a set of measuring spoons. We didn't buy a birthday cake, though, because she is on a diet.

If I tell you this, will you promise not to tell anybody? Okay, guess how much I weigh. I probably weigh way more than Aunt Nada—I weigh 120 pounds. I wrote to Aunt Nada to ask her to send me one of her fabulous diets that really works but I said I just want to be super-slim for the summer. If I told her that I weighed 120 pounds, she'd probably faint.

I feel like I'm eating much more than I used to. My favorite thing for lunch is an "anything you can find in the kitchen between two slices of bread" sandwich. And you know how fattening that can be…

Four months ago, I weighed 108 pounds — I gained 12 pounds! Every day, the scale is going higher and higher… HELP!

Love,
Natasha

And if I could write back to myself, here's what I'd say:

October 20, 2016

Dear young Natasha,

This is your adult self here. I just read the letter that you — er, that I — wrote almost forty years ago and I see you're about to go on your very first diet.

Well, well. I guess that means you're officially a woman. I may have caught you just in time.

As your wiser, older self, I want to gently warn you what is about to happen if you go ahead with it:

You will spend the next three decades going on and off diets. At one point, you'll even pay a doctor to inject you with… cow placenta. Yes, cow placenta, in order to lose weight. Or was it cow urine? I can't remember, but neither sounds good. Around that time, you'll try a 500 calorie-a-day diet before breaking down in tears after four days and wolfing down a Chipwich at 2 A.M. You will think that means you have no willpower (but it doesn't).

You will stop wearing shorts at fourteen because you think your legs are too muscular (but they're not) and stop playing sports *at sixteen for the same reason. You'll wear big, tent-like shirts for years to hide your chest and will waste time reading soul-killing fashion magazines instead of* War and Peace.

And here's the rub: You aren't even overweight! You just have a big, strong, voluptuous build, like your ancestors back in The Old Country. And this first diet, which you don't need, will plop you on an unhealthy road.

Here's the good news:

In about twenty-five years, you will like your unique body type and wear clothes that show it off instead of hiding it. And you'll return to sports, even running The New York Marathon — wearing shorts! (Yes, yes… you will live in Manhattan, your dream city. In a loft! But I digress…).

So please, just skip this first diet you're about to start and take the road that leads directly to the self-acceptance part. Trust me, you will be happier. And you'll get to your New York loft sooner.

Lots of love,

The Future You

~Natasha Stoynoff

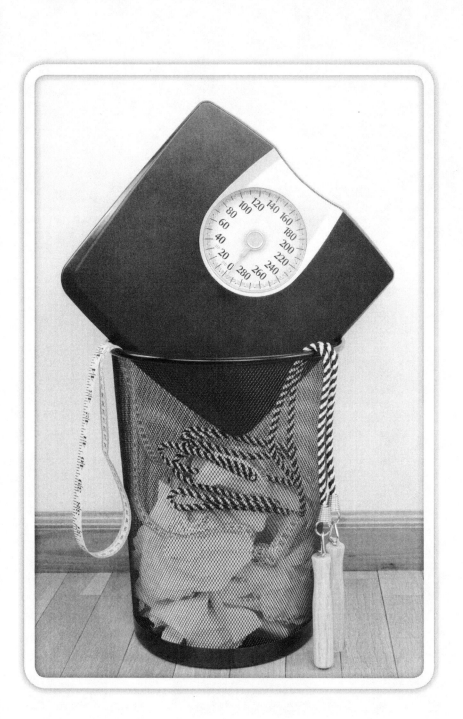

Curvy & Confident

Nourishing My Body

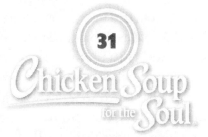
Zen and the Art of Body Maintenance

If you want to conquer the anxiety of life, live in the moment, live in the breath.

~Amit Ray

It's Monday morning and I should probably be at my desk making phone calls by now, but I'm not. I'm lingering in bed, naked and alone, tucked into my linen sheets and basking in the sun from the window.

My To-Do List can wait; this moment and all moments like it are too precious to miss or waste. And I'm in no rush.

There was a time, ten years earlier, when I would have been racing around already, pumped up and frenetic, like a hamster on an endless, spinning wheel — which is how most hard-working women live their lives.

But I don't do that anymore. Cancer was a great teacher to me — perhaps my best teacher so far. It was my wake-up call to slow down, change my pace, and appreciate and love my body more than ever.

I was always tall and strong, an athlete who excelled at hiking, biking, rowing, and snowshoeing. I was curvy and fleshy, too, which was not looked upon kindly by my stepfather. When I was thirteen, he made me stand in front of him in my underwear and, with a black magic marker, he drew on my body — giant, dark circles around areas where, he said, I had too much fat and it had to go.

It took time to heal from that memory and learn to accept and love my natural shape, and then even more time to be confident enough to walk the New York runways as a plus-size fashion model.

But the time, perhaps, when I was most proud of my natural physique that my stepfather hated so much was during chemo treatments. I was beyond thankful for my sturdy, strong body and what it was able to fight and how it was able to heal.

> *Cancer was a great teacher to me — perhaps my best teacher so far.*

At my weekly chemo sessions, I'd bound into the chemo room bustling with energy and pink-cheeked from the healthy, raw green drinks I was downing by the quart. The doctors and nurses couldn't believe — or understand — how healthy I looked and acted when all their other patients in the room were sleepy and ashen-faced as the chemo chemicals were pumped into their bodies.

"Whatever you're doing," they'd say, "keep doing it."

Had I been much thinner, weaker and more fragile, I was told, I would not have withstood the chemo as I did or rebounded as quickly as I did after each session.

During chemo is when I began the practice of meditation.

My "fast forward" button was broken and "pause" was my new speed. I needed to slow myself down to conserve energy for healing, and it felt so good I never stopped.

Before I go onto the red carpet (or, "walking the plank" as some call it) at an event, I do a little meditation-visualization exercise: I visualize light all around me and bathing me, so that when I walk down the carpet and into the event, I can radiate love and peace.

Today, I meditate every morning for twenty minutes as soon as I get out of bed — and for one hour on weekends. It's when I get all my creative ideas for clothes I want to design or books I want to write. It pauses me and keeps me in the present moment.

Which today, is lounging in bed. I take the time to appreciate my curves and pay them honor because they help me climb mountains, they got me a college scholarship, they gave me a career, and they saved my life. *Thank you* sturdy hips, fleshy stomach, wide shoulders and strong legs; all the areas that were marked black and bad by my stepfather have now been powerfully reclaimed as my most beautiful assets.

After fifty-three years of being on this earth, I can take this little me-appreciation-break without feeling any guilt or pressure to hurry up and get somewhere or do something for someone else.

My phone calls can wait. But this lovely moment cannot.

~Emme

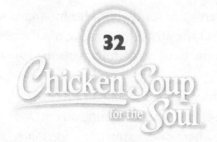

32

An Iron Mother

*I am beginning to measure myself in strength, not
pounds. Sometimes in smiles.*
~Laurie Halse Anderson

The fitness room at the Holiday Inn in Fort Lauderdale
has two treadmills, one loud StairMaster, two station-
ary bikes, neatly rolled white towels by the door, and a
very commanding doctor's scale.

As I spin and sweat on the bike, the smiling woman next to me
steps off the treadmill with relief. Ten minutes later she comes back,
this time in her bathing suit to use the scale. The least amount of
clothing is obviously very important.

She rushes out as a blond woman in Spandex dashes in. "Just
checking my weight!" the blond woman explains, as if apologizing for
coming and going so quickly.

A woman's relationship with the scale is complicated. I no longer
own one and haven't had one in our home for twenty years. When
my son was little he stretched out a tape measure and said, "Mommy,
I know you never like to know how much you weigh. Is it the same
for how tall you are?" But over the years, my children have come to
better understand why I needed a clean break.

I began my unhealthy affair with an iron gray scale in my mother's
bathroom at sixteen. It was rusty, cold and very powerful in my world.
It was how I coped, how I cried, how I survived my parents' divorce.

They had fought for years but I managed. When they divorced I didn't manage as well, and instead, the scale began to manage me. She was someone I trusted, she was always there, and her message was clear and unemotional. I could come and go and she'd be there when I returned, to comfort me and compliment me for being thin.

Soon, however, I was controlled and abused by this iron mother. She wouldn't let go. A pound more, and her imagined criticism made me feel sad, mad, and anxious. A pound less, and I was her proud and confident daughter. Like a film director, she controlled my expression and feeling — and gave me a voice that was not my own.

> *Sometimes I wonder if my children feel deprived that they've grown up without a scale.*

I was a young woman ruled by numbers. But recovery from an eating disorder, with the help of therapy, yoga, spirituality, and my loving family and friends, helped me face the truth about my iron despot. She turned into a piece of metal and I turned into the iron maiden who had the power. One blue-sky morning in Colorado I buried her in a Safeway Dumpster, which seemed like an appropriate farewell.

I know there are many women who can use the scale in a healthy way to monitor their physical health and wellbeing. I am not one of them. It isn't easy to measure myself by weighing my emotions, but it is a safer life raft than holding on to something so heavy it would sink me in the end.

I continue to ask the kind nurse at my yearly check-up not to tell me my weight. "Oh deary you, what's the worry?" she questions.

But, as I recommend to my patients who have a history of abuse, it is up to them what kind of relationship, if any, they want to have with their perpetrator. Sometimes I wonder if my children feel deprived that they've grown up without a scale. But the health of their real mother does seem more important.

So, for now, I prefer to walk on by the ominous creature, celebrating life free from its grasp and appreciating the challenge of finding my own internal "balance." And what did I say to my young son many years ago? "Sure you can measure how tall I am, but the truth is we never stop growing on the inside, so we'll have to find a really big tape measure!"

~Priscilla Dann-Courtney

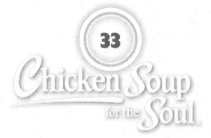

33

Little Girl, Lost and Found

*It takes courage to grow up and become
who you really are.*
~E.E. Cummings

I locked the door behind me in the bathroom stall, pulled down my pants and sat on the toilet. And that's when it happened: my shapewear camisole flipped up while my tummy fell out. It was actually quite comical! But the laugh I stifled in my throat died off as I stared down at my stomach, now resting on my thighs. How had it come to this — my wearing a tight-fitting camisole to hold it all in?

Growing up, I was a confident girl. I was always riding my bike, climbing trees, and building forts. I preferred to play with boys. If anyone gave me a hard time, I was quick to retort, be it with a cheeky comeback or even a decent shove. I could hold my own with anyone. I felt strong and capable.

But at some point, all that changed. Around age twelve, I became aware of different body types. Playing with boys suddenly wasn't as appealing, but I didn't fit in with the girls in my class. They were slender and already wearing make-up. I had an athletic build and didn't have a clue about make-up. I had the sense that I was missing out, as if all the other girls had a secret but I was not a member of the club. They were moving forward, and knew how to do it, while I was standing still. I ached to fit in.

Fast forward several years, and I was married to the love of my life and we had been blessed with two beautiful children. But I was still busy comparing myself to others. Everyone seemed to have self-confidence, while I felt unsure and critical of my body. I still longed to feel like the confident child I used to be. How would I get back to that place?

I realized that part of my problem with self-confidence was my weight. Having had two babies, plus a plethora of poor food choices and very little exercise, meant that I had watched the scale go up and down, and then go up and stay there. It wasn't just that I wanted to lose weight — there is diabetes in my family and I was scared that I was on track to developing it, given my lifestyle. At thirty-four years old and 197 pounds, I was not healthy. I was worried about the example I was setting for my children.

> *I still longed to feel like the confident child I used to be.*

I bought a book online which addressed different types of metabolisms. I felt an instant connection with the author; so much of what she was describing resonated with me! I had many of the symptoms she discussed, including carbohydrate cravings and lack of energy. I believed her eating and exercise plan would help me attain my own health. I decided that I would enjoy Christmas and then on the morning of December 26th, I would start my new lifestyle. And so I did!

I revamped my eating habits entirely. No more muffins for breakfast. No more chicken fingers and fries, or two plates of pasta, for lunch or dinner. No more bowls of ice cream for dessert. These items were to be treats, not a daily habit. My eating plan now included grilled chicken, steamed vegetables, salads, nuts and seeds, smoothies, and high fibre breads and crackers — all in proper portion sizes. I cut out fruit juice and increased my water intake. I started walking five kilometres four to five times a week. The scale began to move down. My hard work was paying off!

Eight months after my Boxing Day start, I was 50 pounds lighter! My husband Russ and I went shopping for new clothes for the "new me." I remember picking pants and tops off the rack and asking his opinion. He looked at me with a smile and said, "That's your OLD size. Let's find you something in your NEW size." I frowned, looking down at the clothes in my arms. What was wrong with me? After all my hard work, I still didn't feel like I deserved a smaller size.

Here's the trouble: I was new on the outside, but not on the inside. My mind needed to catch up to my body, but how? I wanted to find that confident, feisty little girl inside of me. What had made me feel good about myself when I was younger? I couldn't put my finger on it.

It was some time later that I was walking on our treadmill in the basement and suddenly had the urge to start running. I'm not a runner, and had always assumed I just couldn't do it. But something made my finger press the buttons and the belt sped up faster and faster… and suddenly, I was running! Five minutes passed, then ten minutes and the next thing I knew, I had been running for fifteen minutes straight! I was literally shrieking with joy!

It wasn't long before I ventured outside to run. I initially felt awkward and self-conscious, but as I kept going, my attention shifted to my breathing, my heart rate and how my muscles felt. The blood rushing through my veins made me feel alive! I felt strong and purposeful. *Well, hello there, little girl! Welcome back!*

The following year, I signed up for a charity 5K run. Standing there at the starting line, I began to compare myself to the other runners. Then I gave my head a shake; the only person I was competing with was myself. There were going to be runners in front of me, and runners behind me. And that was okay. I wasn't going to worry about anyone else. When I crossed the finish line, I felt amazing. The following year, my goal was to beat my time from the previous year. And I did!

When I look at my daughter Julia, who is seven years old, I am reminded of myself as a little girl. Julia is whole; there are no cracks in her confidence. She loves to ride her bike and climb trees. She is healthy, strong and confident. Julia is beautiful! I want Julia to love her athletic build, just like I learned to love mine, and to feel good about herself. If she ever has doubts, I will help her rediscover the things that make her feel her personal best.

Close your eyes, and think back to your childhood and the things that made you feel confident and beautiful. Find that little girl inside of you. You go, girl!

~Carole Johnston

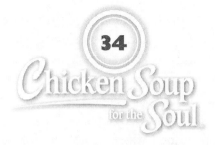

34

In This Moment

Love yourself first and everything else falls into line.
You really have to love yourself to get anything
done in this world.
~Lucille Ball

When I was fourteen, my first boyfriend called me pleasantly plump. He'd hug me and say, "There's just more to love on you."

When I was sixteen, my dad nicknamed me "Thunder Thighs."

Another boyfriend, when I was twenty-two, asked if I was pregnant because I'd gained so much weight.

Needless to say, their words made me feel unloved, judged and insecure.

So I would try to show my love for myself through food. I never attained satisfaction though, and the pounds piled on like a protective layer between the rest of the world and me.

My pride kept me trapped for years, hiding behind baggy tunics and stretchy pants. I'd tell myself, "I'm pretty cool, wearing fancy yoga pants every day." But who was I kidding? I hadn't done yoga in years. Stretchy pants were the only fabric I could squeeze into.

If only I could lose 10 pounds, I thought, *I'd be happy and my life would be great.* That 10 pounds turned into 20, 30, and then 50. For years I tried to change my body, forcing myself to endure uncomfortable diets and distasteful cleanses while suffocating in guilt because I couldn't keep the weight off or keep the cookie dough at bay. I'd squeeze my fat and cry, begging God to grant me a skinny body. But even when I did lose weight, I didn't feel comfortable in my own skin.

I pushed away men I was interested in because I was ashamed of my body. I passed up social engagements to protect myself from judgment and criticism of my weight.

My addiction to food was the problem, or so I thought. Why couldn't I be a normal person around food? Why did I shove food in my mouth when I wasn't even hungry? Why couldn't I put the peanut butter down?" I'd try to answer those questions every day, after each new food binge, but the answers eluded me.

For the past twenty-five years it's been me against my body — a painful, insecure, self-defeating battlefield.

A few months ago I said to a friend, "I weigh more than I ever have, I'm in the largest pants size of my life." The elastic was cutting into my stomach, but I was too stubborn to admit I needed a larger size.

A few days after that, I saw a quote that hit me to my core: "Accept what you can't change and change what you can't accept."

I realized that if I couldn't change myself, then maybe the real issue was one of self-acceptance. After years of sacrifice and suffering, my only other choice was to accept what I couldn't change. Gulp. Could I actually look in the mirror and like what I saw, even with stretch marks and 50 extra pounds cushioning my body? Could I completely love myself despite my body? From that day forward, I made this my full-time mission.

I started to approach food differently. Instead of saying I couldn't have something, I told myself I could eat whatever I wanted as long as I enjoyed it fully. This meant really tasting it — embracing the texture, the flavor, even taking in the smell. Instead of obsessing over what I ate or counting the calories in my chewing gum, I loosened the reins. I accepted that I really do love food, which led me to the real miracle — accepting myself.

Soon, I wasn't hiding or being ashamed of myself. I began to acknowledge that my body is a vessel for love and that I have a lot of love to give to the world. So the bigness I exhibit is a desire to be seen and give my heart to the world.

I began repeating the mantra, "I accept myself in this moment. I am right where I need to be. I am beautiful and full of life."

At first I didn't believe this, but in time I was able to retrain my brain to see the good. And as I embraced myself, I returned to my true self.

Once I admitted that I really like sugar and that eating it makes me happy, my cravings diminished. I stopped wanting it because I knew I could eat it whenever I wanted. My desire to shove cookie dough in my face has gone away. I replaced my years of resistance and pushing away the foods I loved with a more compassionate approach: consciousness.

> *Now I eat what I want when I want.*

Now I eat what I want when I want. I make healthy choices and feel more grounded. Accepting my desires has changed my life.

My shift was simple; I turned down my mind and tuned into my heart. Instead of trying to reach a predetermined idea of perfection, I turned inward. The result? Freedom and self-awareness. No more body hate and no more self-sabotaging thoughts.

With my obsessive food thoughts gone, my body is returning to a healthy weight.

All because I stopped fighting myself and embraced the real me, the one who loves life fully and enjoys each moment, even when... no, especially when... she's eating chocolate cake!

~Shannon Kaiser

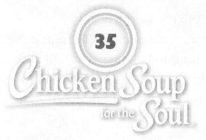

A Blessing, Not a Curse

If you're happy, if you're feeling good, then
nothing else matters.
~Robin Wright

I listened as the oncologist reviewed the stats from my last visit. "White blood cells are looking good. Blood pressure is back to normal. Oxygen has improved. Your weight —"

"I know, it's still high," I interrupted, interpreting his furrowed brow as disapproving.

This wasn't the first time I was about to receive a lecture on my size. For the past twenty years, despite all my efforts, my weight only increased — with a few exceptions. Cancer was one of them.

Before I was officially diagnosed I had lost my appetite, specifically for sweets (my main downfall), and dropped almost 10 pounds. I thought it was a miracle my sweet tooth had been cured. Until the pain came and tests revealed my tumor, which explained my lack of appetite.

Now, thanks to chemo, I was down 25 pounds. But I knew that at 5' 1" and 160 pounds, I was still considered heavy. I was doing my best to be as healthy as possible, but…

"I don't understand. I'm barely eating. Even when I manage to get something down, I throw it back up. I can't get my weight to go any lower," I complained, defeated.

Because that's what I felt I was, concerning my weight: totally beaten. I'd been on restricted calorie diets over the years and if I was lucky, I lost a couple of pounds here and there. But I'd never been on a "diet" like the chemo regime of the past three months. It was a good day if I could eat a couple of canned pears and maybe one scrambled egg and keep it down. Yet, while I had lost weight, I still wasn't losing it easily.

"Lower?" Dr. Patton said. "Oh no, you don't want to lose any more weight. Don't try to do that. Your weight is fine. Leave that alone."

Wait. What?

No doctor had ever said those words to me before. I expected to be admonished like I had been every other time about my weight.

"That's what's helping your fight," his nurse explained, clearly seeing my confusion.

"That's what your body is using for its fuel right now," Dr. Patton said. "Don't try to take that away. It can lead to complications."

I started crying.

The nurse, who was built like me, put a comforting arm around my shoulder.

"I know we're always hearing how bad fat can be for health, and, like anything, too much can be bad. But in some cases, like this, fat is good. It comes in handy when your body is in starvation mode. People who are normal weight or too thin often end up having problems like organ failure during chemo. Their body has nothing to fight with. This is when it's good to be a big girl."

I ended up losing a total of 30 pounds during treatments. I had high hopes of maintaining the weight loss afterward.

I had always been physically active, even before cancer. That had never been one of the causes of my being heavy. Bad food choices and sweets were the main culprits. I also favored pizza, cheeseburgers and mac and cheese. Basically, I was a sucker for any high-fat, high-calorie comfort food.

After cancer, I resumed my exercise routine and even added in some new things. I watched my calories and what I ate, but was dismayed when I'd regained 15 pounds in less than a month.

A couple of months later, I was upset that I had pretty much gained back *all* the weight I'd lost, despite improving my eating habits.

Stumped, my primary care doctor tested my thyroid. Normal. She told me to try exercising harder.

> *The only number I need to see is the one on the calendar that lets me know I'm alive to experience another day.*

A month or so later, my three-month oncology checkup was approaching and I was nervous. Hopefully scans would reveal the tumor was still inactive. But I was also nervous that this time my weight might prove an issue.

As I'm prone to do during times of stress, I turned to my journal. Venting my feelings always helped. Before I wrote, I decided to re-read some of the entries I made during my difficult chemo periods. Maybe if I reminded myself how far I'd come, it would make me feel better.

That's when I found an entry I'd forgotten about, one I'd written after the visit when my oncologist said to stop trying to lose weight.

If I beat this and live, I won't ever worry about my weight again. Because I'm alive. And my size helped facilitate that. If I'd been skinny, I might be dead right now.

These days, I'm back to my pre-cancer weight. However, I'm even more active than I was pre-cancer. I play tennis, walk, and do yoga, each multiple times a week. From blood sugar and cholesterol to blood pressure and thyroid, my stats are all good. I may not look like society's idea of healthy, but my numbers say I'm fit.

On days when I feel down about not dropping weight, I remind myself that my fat kept me alive when I needed it the most. It was a blessing, not a curse. As long as it doesn't inhibit me from doing the activities I love, what's the issue?

Living is the issue, not the number society says my scale should read. I was always trying to lose weight to reach some magic number that would... what? I'm not sure what I thought it would get me. Other than clothes in a smaller size, I had everything: a loving marriage, friends, a beautiful home, happiness, and most important — health.

So I've abandoned the pursuit for a leaner body. I watch what I eat, because that makes me feel good. So does exercising.

But these days I don't bother weighing myself. The only number I need to see is the one on the calendar that lets me know I'm alive to experience another day.

~Courtney Lynn Mroch

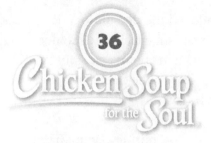

36

The Tutu

People often say that "beauty is in the eye of the beholder," and I say that the most liberating thing about beauty is realizing that you are the beholder.

~Salma Hayek

The tutu fit too tight on my hips. The frilly pink tulle hugged my curves, accentuating the soft tummy protruding over the fabric.

I was drowning in waves of self-consciousness as I padded onto the stage. My feet dragged and time slowed. I couldn't concentrate on the routine our dance instructor had drilled into our heads because I was too distracted by how I must look in my pink leotard. I felt enormous and embarrassed.

I was four.

It's amazing what moments impact a young mind. I can't remember the name of my dance instructor or what we performed or the faces of the girls next to me. But the memory of that shame is vividly etched in my mind twenty-six years later.

That was the beginning of my body image issues.

Assured it was only baby fat and it would melt away, I buried those feelings of shame, until the unthinkable happened. In middle school, I went from only thinking I was the dreaded "f" word to actually *becoming* it.

I began packing on the pounds. Food became a crutch, a way to avoid addressing feelings. Time passed and soon I was in high school and then graduating from college. The evidence of my addiction — stretch marks — spread across my body like roads on a map. I had rolls where I'd never noticed them before and new parts of me rubbed together.

Society didn't help.

There's nothing like someone heckling you from a car window or a child asking if you're going to have a baby to sink your self-esteem faster than an anchor in shallow waters. I'm ashamed to admit, I loved myself a little less.

The turning point was unexpected, as many good things in life are.

I joined a weight loss program focused on healthy living. Figuring that if I loved my body more, then maybe I would love myself more, too. I discovered my mentality was backward — the problem wasn't my body or food, the problem was *me*.

> *Losing or gaining weight wouldn't make me happy — only I could do that.*

It happened during a weekly weigh-in. Buoyed by weeks of consistent weight loss and feeling slim, sexy and confident, I nonchalantly stepped on the scale.

Four pounds. I had gained a whopping 4 pounds.

I frantically reviewed my food choices for the week, obsessing over the burger I'd snuck in between fruit smoothies and meals that featured more broccoli than meat.

I tuned out the meeting, lamenting the voluptuousness of my body and wondering how I could ever learn to love a body with more curves than a Grand Prix racetrack.

In my mind, I was still the little girl in a too-tight pink tutu.

Somehow, a voice broke through my wallowing.

The meeting leader was sharing the story of a woman who had attended 100 meetings and lost 100 pounds. Of the meetings she attended, more than half of those times she lost nothing. Sometimes, she gained weight.

A light bulb went off in my head and I began to see myself in a new light. Losing or gaining weight wouldn't make me happy — only I could do that. And while a scale could be a useful tool, I couldn't let it determine how I felt about myself.

When I asked people why they loved me, no one had ever said anything about my weight. So why was I basing my self-worth on a number?

The scale is a fickle friend and weight is a fluid thing, but the one constant that should always be a solid in your life is your confidence in yourself.

It's ironic, but after thirty years of hating my body, it took gaining weight to help me love it.

~Ashley M. Slayton

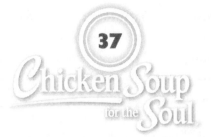

37

Running for My Life

It's the fire in my eyes, and the flash of my teeth. The
swing in my waist, and the joy in my feet.
I'm a woman phenomenally.
~Maya Angelou

A plaque with the silhouette of a city skyline hangs proudly on a wall in my house. Six medals dangle from its hooks, each with a different size, shape, color, and meaning. The one in the middle, though, is my favorite — its thick red ribbon holds a pendant of a buffalo, with the words "Buffalo Half Marathon" and "FINISHER" embossed on it.

Every time the medal catches my eye, I smile and feel unstoppable.

My body and I have known each other for twenty-five years, but we just recently fell in love. Growing up, I was never much of an athlete. While I dabbled with sports and exercise, I had little natural talent and enjoyed junk food far too much.

My family kept sweets, snacks, and soda on hand at all times, and maintained a weekly tradition of indulging at the local pizzeria. As a result, I developed an unhealthy relationship with food. I oscillated back and forth between binging and starving, being sedentary and exercising on an empty stomach.

These habits caught up to me after graduating from college. I'd reached my heaviest weight and my lowest self-confidence. Entering graduate school, I was depressed and resigned to unhealthiness.

My mother had been diagnosed with diabetes several years prior, and each time I watched her test her blood sugar, my stomach grew queasy. Was I looking at my future? I knew something had to change, I just didn't know how to do it. When I looked in the mirror, my stomach would seize at the sight of my thick waistline, thunderous thighs, and jiggly arms. It was like looking in the mirror at a repulsive stranger whom I had no intention of getting to know.

Learning to love yourself in a society that tells you what you are supposed to be is one of the hardest tasks women face, but it is also one of the most urgent jobs we have, especially as women of the next generation. Looking back at pictures from my teens and college years, I realize that I had never actually been overweight. Hating my body, however, had been a theme in my life from a very young age.

> *We were a community of women, and someone had to take the first steps.*

During their adolescence, nearly every woman in my family struggled with an eating disorder, but no one talked about it. My mother and I eventually shared our stories, and as it turned out, they were hauntingly similar, as were my grandmother's and my sister's. I felt a sense of reassurance knowing that it wasn't just me who struggled. We were a community of women, and someone had to take the first steps.

So, I did. Little by little, I started working out here and making a healthy choice there. When I was feeling exceptionally ambitious, I would lace up my sneakers and jog around the block. The next week, I'd jog a little farther, and the next, I'd run.

At first, a little voice in my head whined and told me I couldn't do it. But the longer we ran together, the more we got to truly know one another.

I eventually learned that the little voice didn't really believe I couldn't do it; she was just afraid of failing and falling into old habits. Deep down, she wanted this as much as I did.

After a long talk with a close friend of ours, that little voice and I decided to tackle a seemingly insane task: running a half marathon.

As we embarked on a training routine, she would chime in with her fits of self-doubt, and I would gently talk her off the ledge with chants of "Just a little bit farther!" or "Trust me, we can do this!"

Occasionally, she would call me that ugly three-letter "f" word, even though our waistline was shrinking and our legs were getting leaner and more muscular. I learned to silence her with — of all things — a cookie, because I discovered that depriving her of cravings only made her grow cranky and tiresome. The key was to supplement those treats with whole grains, fruits, and vegetables and to pay close attention to how much I was consuming. Diet is crucial when running thirty-plus miles a week. To work in unison and to make the training program work, that little voice and I needed balance.

Those grueling miles and long weeks of training helped me understand the importance of listening to my body. When my mind told me to stop, it could usually be attributed to doubt, fear, and insecurity. When my body told me to stop, however, it acted as a warning signal against injury, undernourishment, and overexertion.

Before running, I ignored the whispers that came from my body, but once I started running regularly, I listened for them with the attentiveness of a mother awaiting her baby's cry. Sometimes I would disregard them, knowing that my mind was trying to speak for my body, but other times, I would respect my body's wishes and cut back on my mileage or eat a little extra.

I completed my training, and one warm day in May, I crossed the finish line in front of hundreds of spectators, alongside one of my dearest and most encouraging friends. When a happy stranger knighted me with my shiny buffalo, I was exhausted, but my mind was calmer than it had ever been before. After victory photos and post-race snacks, my friend looked at me and smiled.

"You look super athletic, by the way. You've lost weight."

I returned his smile. Covered in layers of sweaty clothing, wearing my first medal, I realized how little those words meant. Together, my body, mind, and spirit stood united and strong; stronger than they had ever been before. To me, that was more beautiful than any compliment.

Now, whenever I feel my confidence waning, I look at my first medal, lace up my sneakers, and remind myself that I run this life.

~Jenna Schifferle

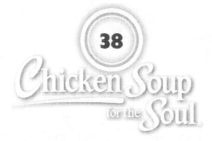

38

The Mirror Girl

Anorexia is an awful thing, but you get yourself into it,
and only you can get yourself out of it.
~Celia Imrie

"Ugh. Look at that flab hanging from your arms, and the padded ring circling your hips. Disgusting! And your thighs? You call those muscular? I call it 'you look like you could use forty minutes on the treadmill and a cup of green juice.'"

I muttered insults to the fifteen-year-old girl staring back at me from the mirror. Most of us would never say these comments to another human being, but this mirror girl was hideous. I grabbed a sweatshirt to conceal the uncomely body, inside of which I was stuck.

I reached high school, and self-doubt smacked me every chance that it could. Walking down the dull, blue halls was a nightmare. The pretty girls were getting prettier, the popular girls were radiating with confidence, and the smart girls were just smart. They stood in their groups, confidence pouring from their smiles, laughs, and funny jokes. And there I was, blending in with the lockers. I was a nobody — an unnoticed girl whose body seemed to have undergone an overnight change that left me feeling like a cow. I told myself, *You're not cool enough to hang out with those people. They don't want to talk to you, why would they? You're nothing special.*

The negative self-talk was crushing me. Until I realized that maybe there was a way I could turn this around. Maybe there was a way that I too, could be beautiful, confident, and popular. I hunted for an answer. What did the pretty girls have that I didn't have? Slimness. What did the popular girls have that I didn't have? Slenderness! Skinny was the common thread, the answer to my self-doubt.

At that moment, I put thinness on a pedestal. I idolized every girl, every model, every actress who was smaller than me, and I envied her slim build. My dad always said that our family was big-boned. At that moment, I despised my big bones. So I set out on a quest to satisfy the hunger that I most craved: a thin body. Then I could be happy, confident and beautiful.

> *At that moment, I saw the price that I was paying for thinness, and I realized that price was much too high.*

"Starting today, no more sweets, chips or soda. And you have to exercise, every day."

The mirror girl looked disappointed, but I was satisfied with my decision to transform her into something worth looking at. I refused to eat junk, and I kept a daily log of my calories. I wrote down everything I ate. It gave me peace of mind to know how many calories I had consumed. It determined whether I could eat a meal, or if I had to skip it. Soon, I saw results, and so did others.

"Mal, you lost weight! You look good," they said.

I was ecstatic. People noticed. I couldn't lose my momentum. I had to maintain my strict diet and exercise routine. But soon, things took a downward turn.

It was a Friday night, in February. I could hear the phone ringing. I was hoping in my head that it wasn't for me. My mom picked it up. It was for me. "Hello?" I mustered up what enthusiasm I could. "Hey Mal! It's Hayley. Me, Sophie and Riley are going out to grab a pizza tonight. Would you like to come?" Why were my friends inviting me to partake in food-related activities? I didn't eat pizza anymore.

"I'm sorry Hayley, I told my sister I'd hang out with her tonight. I can't." It was an excuse. Truthfully, I didn't want to tell her that consuming a slice of greasy, cheesy, fattening pizza would be like digging myself into a hole of guilt and regret.

Food had become my enemy.

"That's okay! Maybe next time. Talk to you later."

"Talk to you later." I hung up the phone and went downstairs to my bedroom. I closed the door, and turned to face the mirror girl.

"You could afford to lose some of that belly fat. Your thighs are still huge. If you don't keep working out, those flabby arms are coming back for you!"

The mirror hung on the back of my bedroom door, and there I stayed, locked away from the temptation of food, so that I could reach my ideal of thinness.

One afternoon, my mother took me to a clinic where I met with a doctor, then a dietician. At 92 pounds, I was about 30 pounds underweight. At some point, I was diagnosed with anorexia nervosa. I had never felt more accomplished. My clothes were loose-fitting, my arms were sticks, my stomach was concave, my cheekbones were jagged. I didn't care about the self-starvation; I had molded myself into society's definition of beauty. I looked like the models and the skinny girls; I was there.

But what had I truly accomplished? Was I confident? Beautiful? Happy?

One afternoon, I walked down to my bedroom and caught a glance of the mirror girl. The girl I saw, the reflection, was someone I didn't recognize. She looked hollow, exhausted, and angry. She looked lifeless. Her image made me stop. Was this my idea of perfection? Was this beauty, confidence and happiness? At that moment, I saw the price that I was paying for thinness, and I realized that price was much too high.

I was slipping away as a student, a friend, a sibling, and a daughter. I no longer figure skated—I had given up my passion. I stopped living life because I was too cold, too exhausted, too afraid that I'd miss a workout. I feared food and felt compelled to check the scale every hour to make sure I hadn't gained a pound. I was living a life of obsessive, fearful misery. And worse than harming myself, I was hurting those who cared.

Luckily, my friends and family never stopped supporting me. I am forever grateful for them because otherwise, I don't think I ever would have snapped out of this detrimental cycle. In time, they helped me put body image and food back into perspective. I began figure skating again, and I learned that food would not make me fat, but that it would give me the energy I needed to fulfill my passions and to live life.

Since that period of time, I've never looked at the mirror girl in the same way. I've never insulted her, or hurt her. I decided that from then on, I had to treat this mirror girl with respect. I celebrated her beauty, despite her imperfections; and from this experience I learned one of the most critical lessons about beauty, confidence and happiness. It is that in cherishing our own flaws, imperfections and uniqueness lies our true beauty, and once we embrace ourselves for who we are rather than what we look like, without regard for what others think, do we truly become our most confident and happiest selves.

~Mallory Lavoie

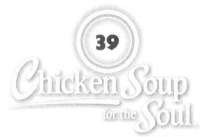

39

No Shame in My Game

Be who you are and say what you feel, because those
who mind don't matter and those who
matter don't mind.
~Dr. Seuss

I looked in the mirror and nodded my head in approval. It was going to be a great day!

I'd recently been invited to help decorate for an upcoming women's retreat at a local church. Sylvia was on the planning committee and when she invited me to do some shopping for the event I eagerly accepted. It would be nice to get out of the house and I looked forward to getting to know this lady better. I wanted to make a good impression on my new "church friend" so I took extra care in my appearance. She arrived and I confidently greeted her at the door.

We agreed we would stop for lunch first, because shopping for tablescapes is serious business and you need your strength. Sylvia suggested Golden Corral, an all-you-can-eat buffet. We arrived and I headed straight for my favorite section — the salad! I loaded my plate with lettuce, cauliflower, and cucumbers.

As I reached for the salad dressing a man bumped into me. "Oh, I'm sorry. Excuse me," I said pleasantly. I hadn't moved so I knew it was he who had bumped into me. He was an older man and I thought that perhaps he'd stumbled. I felt a little sorry for him. I didn't want him to feel bad so I apologized first.

"I guess you just couldn't wait to get to the food, could you?" he answered curtly.

I was rather surprised by his tone but I just smiled and began to ladle on the ranch dressing.

"I mean, look at you," he continued. "Look how *big* you are."

"Just more of me to love," I answered, managing a nervous laugh.

Was this guy for real? As he continued his verbal lashing I had a flashback to a recent Friday night when my husband Joey and I sat on the couch watching an episode of *What Would You Do?* The ABC show, hosted by 20/20 veteran John Quinones, features actors playing out shocking scenes in public and captures the responses of unsuspecting bystanders. We enjoyed the show but some of the scenarios seemed rather far-fetched to me. One such episode featured an actress playing an overweight woman at an all-you-can-eat buffet. The idea was that they would have another actor berate and humiliate her to see how the other patrons would respond. "That would never really happen," I told Joey. "Nobody is that mean." And I believed that statement one hundred percent.

> *"I guess you just couldn't wait to get to the food, could you?"*

Now here I was. Overweight. At an all-you-can-eat buffet. And I was being berated by a stranger who as far as I could tell was *not* an actor.

Okay, John Quinones, you and your camera crew can come out now. This really isn't funny. And by the way, I no longer feel sorry for the old guy.

John Quinones didn't appear and I stood frozen at the salad bar unsure of what to do next. I had ladled so much dressing onto my salad while contemplating my escape from this crazy old coot that I now had ranch soup. I decided to do what any grown forty-year-old woman who is being fat-shamed by a total stranger in public would do — make a run for it. I turned and took several steps away but the old man cut me off, blocking my path. He continued his tirade, his voice loud enough for everyone around us to hear.

"Look at you! You're *fat*!" He practically yelled it as he looked me up and down in a show of disgust. "I'm eighty-four years old and I have never looked like you."

I didn't know what to do or say. I looked down at myself, taking in the body he was so maliciously criticizing. A million thoughts ran through my head. Should I try to shame him by telling him that I had gained weight while suffering from depression after my daughter passed away? Should I try to explain that much of the weight gain had been a side effect of the anti-depressant medications I had been treated with after my loss? Would sharing something so personal quiet his rant? Would it matter to him that I hadn't always looked like this… that I had once been thin? And then it hit me… Did it matter to me?

Sure I had gained some weight, but I had gained something else along the way. I'd become much more compassionate toward other hurting hearts. I had found a sense of peace after surrendering my circumstance to God. I gained perspective and insight into the people and things that are truly important in life. I felt wiser, and I'd venture to say I was a better person than I'd ever been.

I had liked what I saw when I looked in the mirror that morn-ing—a woman on her life's journey. I was finally feeling better after years of grieving my loss, and it felt good to feel good again. I would not allow this man, a complete stranger, to steal my joy.

"You're *fat!*" The old man said it again… in case the kitchen staff hadn't heard him the first time.

I noticed a woman take a step toward us. I looked up and was horrified. It was Sylvia! How embarrassing! She stopped and her mouth dropped open. I looked back and forth from the old man to my new friend as Sylvia's eyes and mouth grew wider with each hateful word the old man spewed at me.

Sylvia took a deep breath and I could tell she was about to say something. She looked mad, too. Good! My new friend was about to come to my rescue and I could tell she was about to let this crazy old bird have it! I waited… And then it came.

"That's not very Christian of you!" she blurted out as she stared the old man down.

I'm not sure what I was expecting her to say but I can assure you it wasn't that. The old man looked at her stunned. He was quiet for the first time in what seemed an eternity. He turned away and quickly disappeared into a far corner of the restaurant.

"Maybe he's senile and he didn't know what he was doing," Sylvia offered sympathetically as I sipped my ranch soup back at our table.

"No, I think he was just a jerk," I responded.

That evening I played the old man's words over and over again in my head. I knew exactly what had caused my weight gain, but what unseen "thing" would cause a person to verbally assault a complete stranger about her physical appearance? For the second time that day, I felt sorry for the old man. He was no more than a bully whose words said more about him than they did about me.

I was not about to let someone else dictate my self-worth, and as simple as it sounds, I let his words go. They weren't really mine to hold on to in the first place.

In the words of the fictional character, Aibileen Clark, in *The Help*: "You is kind. You is smart. You is important." And may I add, "You is beautiful."

~Melissa Wootan

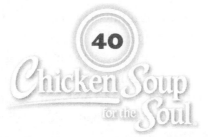

40

My Lovely Lady Lumps

We cannot direct the wind but we can adjust the sails.
~Author Unknown

My breasts. They started growing when I was about eleven. I woke up one morning and felt these funny hard things and thought something was wrong with me.

When I asked my mom what the heck was going on, she smiled with pride and said, "Oh honey, you're starting to *develop*."

Since Judy Blume's book, *Are You There God? It's Me, Margaret.* was the hottest novel among my peers at the time, I breathed a sigh of relief that I was on the fast track to becoming a woman.

Once my breasts began to appear through my T-shirts (with my name ironed on in metallic, rainbow letters circa early-1980's fashion), it was time to get fitted for my first bra. Mom insisted on taking me to a "professional" — an old Russian lady with bifocals and big, scary hands. I'm sure I gasped when she reached toward my new "little lady lumps" to take my measurements.

I vividly remember when a boy touched my breasts for the first time. We had already kissed so I knew "second base" was next. I was scared out of my mind but when it actually happened... well... since my parents will likely read this, let's just say it was a positive experience and leave it at that.

I always had small breasts, but they were pretty and appropriate for my petite frame. They stood as tall as they could in my pretty pink prom dress. And on my wedding day, they were propped up nicely with a beautiful white strapless bra. I nursed both of my daughters with my little lady lumps and loved the bond that created.

As I approached my mid-thirties, my mother strongly encouraged me to get tested for the BRCA breast and ovarian cancer gene. She and several other women in our family had tested positive for it (including her mother, her mother's sister, her cousin... the list goes on). At first, I was apprehensive. But I decided it would be better to know if I had it so I could take the right precautions. I was about thirty-five when I went for the blood test and learned I was positive for the gene and...

> *I was about thirty-five when I went for the blood test and learned I was positive for the gene.*

it sucked, there's no other way to describe it. But at least I knew ahead of time that I was at risk.

Every six months I had either an MRI, a clinical exam, or a mammogram. I felt like I was surrounded by a force field of protection because I was so closely monitored.

Until one day, during an exam, a not-so-nice lump was discovered in my left breast. "I'm sure it's nothing," I said to the nurse, "I just saw my doctor." She gently patted me on the back and sent me off to have my mammogram in the next room.

A biopsy revealed that I did indeed have breast cancer. When the doctor told me, I felt the room spinning around me. As a course of treatment, I chose to get a bilateral mastectomy.

Alas, I had to say goodbye to my lovely lady lumps. When I took my last shower with them I knew I was saying goodbye.

Modern science is pretty amazing. I was told I would wake up from surgery with littler lady lumps. The doctor didn't say it like that; he said I would feel like I had little baby breasts because they would insert a small implant to begin the reconstruction process.

I had to do chemotherapy before I could dive into breast reconstruction. It was definitely a long road, and a long mourning period over the loss of my little lady lumps.

Now, more than three years later, I'm happy to report that my new (not so little) lady lumps are doing just fine. I'm still me.

I have a very slight scar across each of my breasts. At first, when I saw them in the mirror, I hated them and hated what happened to me.

But as time marches on and my survival is evident, I see them as a sign of strength. Like stamps in my passport, they show where I've been.

My little lady lumps. They are still me. They are beautiful.

~Melissa Berry

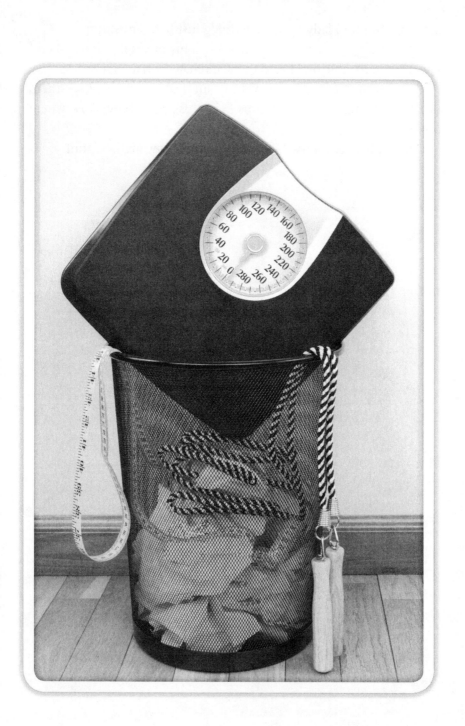

Curvy & Confident

Living Life with Gusto

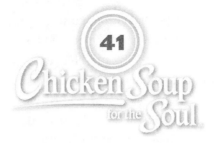
Pork and Beans

The things we hate about ourselves aren't more real
than things we like about ourselves.
~Ellen Goodman

From my earliest memory I knew I was not what I should be. I was not *her*. It wasn't my sister's fault. Just a year and a half older than me, she naturally possessed all the things my father adored in a little girl. She was a skinny little thing with knobby knees, dark hair, olive skin and an impish smile. When she cried, he scooped her up. When her temper flared, he admired her spirit. He called her String Bean.

That was not how he felt about me. He called me Porky.

Maybe it's understandable. I was unplanned and born on a particularly hot summer day when my father was out of work and suffering from considerable depression. Worrying about feeding the family he already had, he had little to offer a new daughter. But even after finances improved and his feelings for me warmed, I grew up knowing I was very different from the little girl he already loved.

My wispy hair was dirty blond. I was fair and freckled, with a tendency to burn. I was stout, too, outgrowing my sister by the age of three, which put me ahead of her in the hand-me-down brigade. When she tried on my old clothes, they slipped right off her narrow hips. "You have no meat on your bones at all!" Dad said with a smile.

I watched and listened, trying to copy my sister's mannerisms, to be dainty and petite instead of big and clumsy. It didn't work and

Dad ridiculed me for my efforts. I tried to bury my hurt, but I kept growing. When I was a teenager, I dieted and fasted. I weighed myself incessantly and started comparing myself to every girl I knew. I took up sports, hoping to slim down. No matter what I did, I never lost weight.

By the time I was an adult I towered over my sister. She had remained skinny and topped out at 5'4". I was an anomaly in my family at 5'9" with arms as thick as her legs. In family pictures, I looked out of proportion — like I had been Photoshopped into the frame.

> *Dozens of pictures — hundreds maybe — passed through my hands that day, showing me a truth that did not match my memory.*

"How did you get so *big?*" people asked me.

Every time I stepped on a scale I felt sick. I knew I should weigh more than she did, but *so* much more? I fantasized about being small — light as a feather — or having a boyfriend who could put his hands around my waist, pick me up and swing me around. He would have a mother who thought I was too skinny and wanted to fatten me up.

Reality was letting me down and I kept gaining weight.

Then one day I was looking through old photographs and found one that struck me. My sister and I were about four and five years old, sitting on our father's knees.

And I wasn't fat.

I started digging through more photos. There I was with my cousin. Not fat. I found another with my mom. Not fat.

Standing next to my sister. Not fat!

Dozens of pictures — hundreds maybe — passed through my hands that day, showing me a truth that did not match my memory. I was never an overweight child. Yes, I was bigger than my sister, but the difference was nothing compared to what I had made it inside my head.

I was dumbfounded. For a long time after that, I thought about the way I felt about myself: my weight, my coloring, my clumsiness, my need to please people — especially my father. I thought about my sister, of whom I had always been jealous. She had grown into a lovely person who had her own issues with our father. And she didn't choose her physiology any more than I chose mine.

Then I thought about my father, who was unkind and critical, but who suffered from life-long depression. Sadly, he remained unhappy with his own life. Was his voice the one I wanted to listen to, to measure my self-worth?

Then I thought about myself—the way I had learned to judge others. I was kind in practice, but in my head I compared myself to every woman I met, thinking: I'm thinner than her, fatter than her, thinner than her, fatter than her...

My father had taught me what beauty was and was not and I had accepted it blindly! I was wasting my youth, yearning for the impossible, caught up in jealousy, destined to fail.

But it didn't have to be that way. I was healthy, with strong arms and legs and a brain that was pretty sharp. My father had let me down, but that didn't mean I had to let him pull me under. I could choose to see myself from a healthier perspective. I could reject the worthless image I had let dominate my mind and rebuild a new one.

I gave up dieting and started focusing on exercise I enjoyed. I started running with a friend and took up Pilates. I made similar changes with food, no longer sneaking high-calorie treats but making conscientious decisions in the light of day. Now I eat right most of the time, cheat occasionally with joy in my heart, and forgive myself when I fail.

More important, I've learned to appreciate my own self-worth. My beauty is as unique as I am, and doesn't need to be compared to my sister or anyone else.

I've also developed a new habit of looking at other women with love and appreciation for their beauty—never as a superficial comparison. It's been eye opening and a complete blessing, because beauty is all around me, in all sizes, shapes and colors. Yet, finally, I am jealous of no one.

I would like to tell you that the change in me was immediate and permanent. That ever since the day I found those pictures, I have never felt bad about my body or freaked out about the number on a scale, but that's not the truth. Everything is a process — a road that goes up and then down again, but one I continue to walk. When bad days creep up on me — days when my father's voice seeps in and mars my self-worth — I remind myself that I forgave him long ago. That letting go of my anger and bitterness is essential to staying positive.

Now, when I look in the mirror, I like what I see. I am not the perfect weight or the perfect size. My skin is not creamy and my hair still needs lots of attention. But the woman who smiles back at me is strong and courageous. She has overcome a difficult childhood and will not pass on those destructive patterns to her own children.

I'm rather fond of her.

~B.J. Dilley

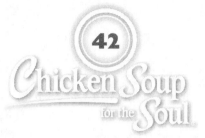

42

A Waist of Tears

If you begin to understand what you are without trying
to change it, then what you are undergoes
a transformation.
~Jiddu Krishnamurti

I was a skinny child — looking as emaciated as those poster children we see in television ads for famine-ravaged countries. I was so thin, my ribs jutted out against my clothing. Everywhere I went, someone felt compelled to offer me food.

Poor as we were, Mom was an amazing cook and could usually stretch what little we had into glorious, mouth-watering meals for our family of six. Dad often said she could take a sock, add some water and spices, and make it taste delicious. We never went hungry.

Being an active and somewhat neurotic child, I burned calories faster than I could absorb them. Apart from three square meals a day, I was a grazer. I would run into the house several times a day to grab a piece of bread with butter, a homemade doughnut, an apple, a handful of freshly picked berries earmarked for jam preserves — anything that happened to be easily accessible. No matter how much I ate, though, I never gained an ounce.

I was a fairly late bloomer, too. Most of my girlfriends were already strutting around in their first training bras while I still looked like a boy from the neck down. The only things that set me apart physically from my three brothers were my long braids and the dresses Mom made me wear.

When I finally entered puberty, you could still see my ribs, but at least I was starting to get a chest. Luckily, it was the 1960's and thin was in. Girls of my generation aspired to look like Twiggy and Pattie Boyd, models who looked so frail that a leashed Chihuahua could have easily dragged them down a street. Suddenly, my body was something my peers envied. The skeletal jokes stopped. Instead, my svelte physique was all the rage.

By my early twenties I had stopped growing vertically, coming to a full stop at an unimpressive five feet, one and a half inches. I towered over Mom by a full three inches, but remained dwarfed by pretty much everyone else on the planet. It was then I began noticing a slight thickening in my hips and waist. My thighs developed tiny, almost imperceptible little dimples that I attributed to the contours of my mattress — until my husband and I invested in a new one. Then the blame went to those delightful single serving lemon pies I had for dessert after most dinners.

> *Middle-aged spreads appeared everywhere on women who were still loved by husbands, whose arms encircled them, their own bellies jutting out noticeably.*

Eventually the pie calories over-inflated my buttocks. I gave them up and started taking evening walks. I bought new outfits, shoving the old ones to the back of my closet for "someday."

Just as that someday arrived and I was able to squeeze back into my favorite pre-pastry jeans, I got pregnant. I gained 67 pounds, most of which remained long after delivery. By the time my son, David, was crawling, my closet had two sets of "someday" clothes that were four sizes apart, and I was still wearing some of my maternity tops to cover my stubborn, unsightly bulges.

Reality struck when I saw myself in pictures at my son's first birthday party. My double chin and muffin top were glaringly evident as I held my baby on my lap to help him blow out his solitary candle. It was time to stop blaming my son for my "baby fat" and do something about my own self-neglect.

For the next two decades, I embarked on a series of fad diets. I counted calories, weighed food, avoided carbohydrates, resisted protein, subsisted on watery soup, shunned dairy products, and fasted. I lost weight, but it returned when I could no longer tolerate the side effects of headaches, rashes, dizziness, indigestion or fatigue.

During this time, I dodged the camera like a poacher hiding from game wardens. I agonized over my appearance, despising my reflection. I felt as if everything I wore draped me like a tent. Black became my favorite color. After all, it hides everything, right? Wrong! In my critical mind, I resembled a mutant rhino with a human face.

One day, before I was about to start yet another weight loss regimen, my husband threw a surprise birthday party for me. Thinking we would just be two couples enjoying a barbecue dinner by our hosts' pool, I opted to wear baggy shorts and a floppy top. We were experiencing a blistering heat wave, but I hadn't owned a bathing suit in years. I wouldn't have worn one, anyway. It would have drawn even more attention to my physical flaws.

To my horror, forty people greeted us instead of two. I was mortified. I wore no make-up, was barelegged, and was sure my exposed arms jiggled with every warm hug I received. I embraced everyone self-consciously, wishing I could slink away, but as the guest of honor, that was impossible. Instead, I relaxed, reminding myself how blessed I was that these people were all there for me.

As my gaze drifted around the yard, I saw my son sneak up behind my friend Jean and push her, fully clothed, into the water. She surfaced, crawled out and tore after him, shrieking with good-natured laughter.

As Jean ran, I noticed that time had not been kind to her once slim body either. Small rolls of skin were visible through her saturated blouse. Her ample chest flopped about with every step, yet her appearance didn't seem to phase her one bit. She was having fun.

Suddenly, I saw everyone around me with new perspective. Middle-aged spreads appeared everywhere on women who were still loved by husbands, whose arms encircled them, their own bellies jutting out noticeably. Female thighs, arms and chins that had once been firm and unblemished showed identical wear, tear, and weight gain to mine. Previously tiny derrieres were sagging, yet deep, defined laugh lines drew attention away from those imperfections. Everyone was simply living life with zest — and they were all here because they cared about me, and not what we all looked like.

A beach ball bounced softly off my head, and I saw my husband grinning at me from the pool. I stood up and did something I hadn't done since my teenage days. I ran toward the pool's edge, jumped as high as I could, and cannonballed into the water right next to him.

"All right, Mom!" I heard my son cry, just as my head went below the surface.

That night, I threw away that last stupid diet book. From then on, I made sensible choices — moderate food portions, water instead of soda, fresh fruit and vegetables as snacks, and some exercise. I also began smiling at cameras.

I didn't lose a lot of weight, and I'm still heavier than I'd like to be, but I'm healthier and more relaxed. I've learned to accept myself the way those I love have always accepted me — flaws and all. Oh, and one more thing — I went out and bought a bathing suit!

~Marya Morin

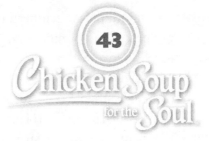

43

The Shell

The greatest happiness of life is the conviction that we
are loved; loved for ourselves, or rather, loved
in spite of ourselves.
~Victor Hugo

It was a freak accident that caused something called a CSF leak in my brain. It was every bit as awful as it sounds. I had to shave part of my head for the surgeries. Surgeries plural. That's right. That's not a typo.

My long, painstakingly and expensively dyed locks were shorn. My body and mind went through extraordinary changes. My once budding filmmaking career was sidetracked while I struggled to walk and feed myself. The most mundane tasks caused tears and frustration.

During this time in and out of hospitals and through the surgeries I went from 5'8" and a 118-pound supermodel body to gaining over 50 pounds. I felt strange and awkward in my own body, like I didn't fit in my skin. I hid. I was ashamed.

Somewhere along the way, during my darkest hours, my best friend fell in love with me. The shaved head, the weight gain, all that stuff was what made me vulnerable, he said. Before, I had been a fierce, career driven woman who didn't give him a second look. Would never have given him a chance. And that fierce woman really looked like she needed to eat a sandwich. Or two. And she didn't look particularly happy, he said.

After the accident he saw me in a different light. And apparently that curvy light suited me, and him. We fell head over heels in love, the whole nine yards. My best friend of nine years who had seen me at my best and brightest fell in love with me when I thought I wasn't lovable anymore, when I felt like a failure.

I'm still 50 pounds heavier than I used to be. But I'm happily married to the man of my dreams. Most days. Some days he's the man I want to kick in the shins. But either way, our marriage and our commitment to each other is unbreakable. He makes me feel like the most beautiful woman in every room.

> *It's about me becoming a more human version of myself, a version that isn't chasing a bizarre ideal.*

And somewhere along the way I realized that I had forgiven my fatter self, forgiven her for becoming someone I thought was below average. I embraced her and changed the way I looked at her in the mirror. I felt beautiful inside and out. And no, it's not a man loving me that changed it. It's about me becoming a more human version of myself, a version that isn't chasing a bizarre ideal.

And it's about realizing that despite the size 0 jeans and the jet-setting across the world I had done before, I was miserable and alone. And I had been so afraid to fail that I had quit being a person.

I now understand why my husband didn't fall for me when I had the body and hair to die for. I was dead inside, only a beautiful shell.

And now the size 12 shell is as full and whole as I could ever dream of being. And I get to eat all the key lime pie I want, on top of it. If that's not the whipped cream and cherry on top of life, I don't know what is.

Embrace yourself and the curves and curveballs life throws at you.

The hardest ones may end up changing everything — for the very best.

~Jennifer Roberts

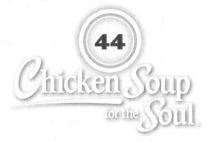

A New Message

You are you. Now, isn't that pleasant?
~Dr. Seuss

"After we're done grocery shopping, can we get a hot pretzel?" my thirteen-year-old daughter, Julia, asked. I sighed. I knew the question was coming — and the temptation that came along with it.

"I'd be happy to buy you a pretzel, Jules, but I'm not going to get one for myself," I said.

Her mouth dropped open. "But you love Ben's hot pretzels dipped in cheese!" she said. "You always say it's the best part about grocery shopping at this store."

"I know, honey. I do love them, but I'm not going to eat one this time."

"Because of your diet?"

I nodded. "Yes. I've lost 9 pounds, and I'd like to lose 10 more. But I can't do it eating hot pretzels dipped in cheese sauce."

"We can share one," Julia suggested, with a shrug.

"That's okay, honey. I don't need the carbs."

"But they're your favorite. Can't you splurge a little?"

"I'll splurge after I reach my goal weight."

We finished shopping, then headed for the hot pretzel stand. My mouth watered as I ordered Julia's treat. We sat down at a table and Julia tore off a piece of her pretzel. I could tell she was about to offer

Living Life with Gusto | 161

it to me, so I shook my head quickly.

As she ate, she filled me in on what was happening at school and with her friends. Our conversation turned to social media.

"Do you remember a Disney show called *Shake It Up*?" she asked. "I used to watch it all the time."

I nodded. "Yeah. About two teenage girls who were on a dance show?"

"Right," Julia said. "Well, one of the girls from the show, Zendaya Coleman, is getting pretty famous. She recently got mad because a magazine Photoshopped pictures of her."

"Why did she get mad? I thought Photoshop made people look better?"

"That's the problem, Mom. The magazine edited her hips and thighs to make her look thinner, but she is already thin enough. She got mad because she thought the magazine was saying that the real Zendaya wasn't good enough."

Julia pulled out her iPhone and Googled the photos, then handed me the phone.

There were two images of Zendaya. One was the original and the other was the edited version. As I compared the two, I felt queasy.

Julia used her finger to point out the obvious: "See how they edited out a bit of fat on her thigh right there and how her hip doesn't jut out at all in this picture?"

I nodded. "Jules, you're right. There is absolutely nothing wrong with the original picture. She is a beautiful girl and I can see why she was upset that the magazine did this."

"Scroll down, Mom," Julia said. "There's a quote from Zendaya. She says that by editing her photo, the magazine was sending the wrong message to young girls and creating unrealistic ideals about how we should look."

I did as Julia asked. I read the words from nineteen-year-old Zendaya about the edits to her photo. She encouraged women to love themselves unconditionally and not to buy into impossible beauty standards.

"She released the real, unedited picture herself, Mom. She didn't want to be a part of making women feel not good enough about their bodies."

"She is a smart girl," I said. "And she sounds like a great role model." As I uttered the words "role model," I felt queasy again. What was wrong with me? Here I sat, praising a teenager for being real and loving her body as it was, while I beat myself up over my extra pounds and made it crystal clear to my daughter that good enough meant thin enough.

I was part of the problem.

"Jules, I owe you an apology," I said, teary-eyed. "Zendaya is right. We should love ourselves no matter what size jeans we wear. Being thin doesn't equal being happy, and it doesn't make us more worthy of love. There are many different ways to be beautiful, but Hollywood rarely shows us that."

> *"She released the real, unedited picture herself, Mom. She didn't want to be a part of making women feel not good enough about their bodies."*

Julia smiled and nodded.

"I need to work on accepting myself as I am and be more careful with the messages I send you."

I grabbed a large piece of her pretzel, dunked it into the cheese sauce, and bit into it, grinning.

"How's that for a new message? I've eaten healthy all day and now I'm going to splurge. Because I love myself and we all deserve a treat sometimes."

"You know what would send an even better message, Mom?" Jules said, smiling. "If you got your own pretzel!"

I hopped up and ordered a second pretzel. As I ate every last bit of it, I didn't think about the calories.

I simply enjoyed the treat — and my daughter's company.

~Diane Stark

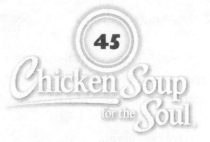

45

Judge Me by My Size, Do You?

*Judge me if you want, but at the end of my life I choose
to have memories not regrets.*
~Steve Maraboli

The two fitness company reps sitting by the promotional display didn't look up from their phones when I said hello. I was at a health and fitness expo held in conjunction with a 5K race I was running. The convention center ballroom was filled with booths and tables advertising everything from sports drinks to other running events. However, I didn't seem to be the customer they wanted.

I moved on to another booth, where they were promoting a holiday 5K race. I picked up a flier and tried to engage the rep in conversation.

"I'm interested in —" He cut me off without even looking at me and shouted over my head at the crowd behind me, inviting them to visit the booth. I put the brochure down and walked away.

I went to the next booth, where a company offered to take free photos of race participants with silly props. I approached the photographer with a smile, but was greeted with indifference.

"What do you want?" He was amazed that I wanted to get my picture taken.

I was frustrated. Walking in 5Ks was an integral part of my life. I completed more than ten organized 5K events every year, medalled in two race-walking 5Ks, and walked miles on my own every week. Even when I became disabled after being diagnosed with several medical conditions, I continued walking and dancing as much as I could. I wasn't as fast and the races left me exhausted for days, but I crossed the finish line of every 5K I entered.

But as far as these exhibitors were concerned, I was invisible. When they did see me, many assumed it was my first race or I received patronizing comments like: "Good for *you*, trying to do a 5K!"

Last fall, I was getting dressed to attend yet another expo and choosing a shirt to wear. I had a huge collection of 5K T-shirts from previous races. I was about to pick up a favorite red one, when I noticed another in my closet — a shirt I'd purchased at Disneyland. It was a *Star Wars* shirt with a single sentence printed on it: "Judge me by my size, do you?" In *The Empire Strikes Back*, Yoda posed this question to Luke Skywalker, who had treated him with derision because of his short stature.

> *But as far as these exhibitors were concerned, I was invisible.*

I felt like I was facing a similar situation when I was judged by my weight. Some people wrote me off the moment they saw me, assuming I couldn't be athletic because I was heavyset, and that I was not worth the same respect and consideration they gave to other people.

I didn't feel comfortable confronting my critics directly, but maybe I could let my shirt speak for me. I put it on, tied my hair back to make sure my message was visible, and went off to the expo.

The difference was drastic and immediate: instead of ignoring me, the shirt became a conversation starter for many vendors.

"That's a very powerful statement," observed one rep, as I strolled into her booth. Another spent ten minutes discussing his event with me. The reps at the sports nutrition booths gave me the same consideration as the thinner race participants standing there. None of them assumed it was my first 5K.

I left the expo with my head held high and a bag full of swag.

Perhaps the other reps and vendors hadn't realized they were showing size bias. Perhaps they knew they were, but didn't care. Either way, Yoda had helped gently remind them that I, and other curvy and heavyset runners and walkers, were worthy of the same respect as everyone else.

I now wear my Yoda shirt to race expos, fitness conventions, dance events, and any other place I may be judged by my size.

It never fails to attract attention, and it always makes people consider their words and behavior toward people of different physiques.

Hopefully, that mindfulness stays with them long after the race is over.

~Denise Reich

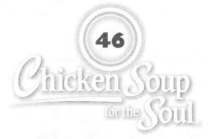

46

Storm

*The great and glorious masterpiece of man is to
know how to live to purpose.*
~Michel de Montaigne

"Should you eat that?" "You shouldn't wear that." "Are you sure you can fit?" "She should exercise." "Put her in sports." "Try a bigger size." These words had echoed in my ears since I was old enough to understand. They became my inner voice.

Should I wear that? I'm too big to do this. Maybe I shouldn't. I can't. Words became action; action became more eating. More eating became a bigger waistline. A verbally abusive partner solidified the deal.

Daily, I was told how beautiful I would be if I were smaller.

I was told that I couldn't be happy unless I was thin.

I waited for happy; it never came. Insane dieting, a divorce, and a fiancé who flew the coop when I was six months pregnant put me in the darkest place of my life.

And at my heaviest — 330 pounds.

One day I woke up. I was holding my three-week-old in my arms and I decided then and there: I was good enough. I was worth it. This tiny person would grow without those words in *his* head.

Did I lose the weight? Not really.

But I did go back to school when my son was three months old.

I did apply for every scholarship I could get my hands on and every bit of financial aid I qualified for. When I didn't fit behind the desks, I sat at the teacher's aide desk. I studied. I passed. I got into nursing school.

I passed nursing school at 320 pounds.

I was on my feet twelve-plus hours a day and went to classes most of the week. I took care of a child at home. I found a way to pay for college.

I worked as a nursing assistant while I waited to pass my boards. I passed.

I got a job at a long-term care facility taking care of fifty-four patients per night.

> *I was told that I couldn't be happy unless I was thin.*

I worked six days a week for months until I got a job at a Long Term Acute Care where I had nine patients a night for twelve-hour shifts. I've been there a year and a half. I never sit.

I was still 310 pounds.

I returned to writing, one of my passions. I spent my nights off staring at a computer screen and writing when everyone else was asleep. I've returned to school to work on my bachelor's degree online. I finished sixty-three hours of critical care training in a month-long weekend class schedule with a full-time job and a kid. I sleep three to five hours a night most nights.

I was still 305 pounds.

I work out. I eat better. It's a learning process. But I don't have to be thin to be strong. I don't have to be thin to be happy. I have a beautiful, energetic and hilarious son, a promising and fulfilling career, a rewarding hobby, and a loving family. I found my happy. I found myself.

I accepted a new position at a magnet hospital in their ICU.

I'm still 300 pounds.

Curvy is not a complete roadblock to being you. I still shimmy and dance in Storm Trooper scrubs. I do everything I set out to do. I'm getting to a healthier me but I don't let words stop me from wearing a dress, going out or living my life.

The words I hear now are mine. *I am good enough. I am worth it.*

So are you. You have always been good enough. You have always been worth it. You do not need to rely on anyone for your happy. You are strong, stronger than you know, and you can do anything.

Say that, repeat daily. Then take the world by storm.

~Jillian Rossi

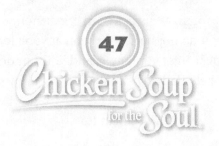

47

Tunnel of Love

When a child is born, so are grandmothers.
~Judith Levy

"Levi, go get your daddy!" I implored my three-year-old grandson. Off he ran, his tiny bare feet slapping the wood floor. I cringed a bit as I heard him holler to my son-in-law: "Grandma 'tuck!" I squirmed a bit as I listened to Johnny's approaching footsteps, and forced a smile as Levi came back into view. He pointed a tiny finger at me.

Grandma was indeed stuck. It was completely my own fault. Levi and I had been engaged in a jolly game of hide-and-seek. We'd taken turns hiding. He was always easy to find. He'd cover his head with a corner of the rug and consider himself well hidden. Or he'd wriggle under his bed, leaving his toes vulnerable to a tickling when I'd find him. I have my usual places to hide: behind the shower curtain, the couch or the laundry room door. But today I had spotted a new place to try! Levi had a springy play tunnel that he loved to crawl through. My good judgment took a temporary break as I slithered into it like a snake. My upper body fit well; it was my mid-section that met resistance. Somehow, I was able to wriggle most of myself in and patiently waited for Levi to find me.

It didn't take him long since it was a 5' tunnel and I'm a 5'4" grandma. He giggled with excitement, shouting, "I found you!" I laughed with him and declared him a clever boy, indeed. It was time to exit, so I began to wiggle my way forward. I advanced an inch or two but my hips seemed to be wedged. I decided to back out. I put more vigor into my wiggle, twisting with all my might. Levi sat down cross-legged to watch the show.

I could not get out. Since I had entered face first and worm-like, my arms were trapped at my sides. Red-faced and damp with exertion, it was then that I had sent Levi for help.

At first, Johnny stood speechless. What do you say to a pair of adult feet sticking out of a child's toy? He walked around to the other end and peered in. I could clearly see the smirk that he was trying to hide.

"Don't ask questions; just help me out!" I said.

What followed was probably the most comical fifteen minutes of my life. Since he couldn't pull or push me, he somehow managed to get both the tunnel and me into a standing position. That part is a blur. I do remember chanting a prayer. From that point, he slowly eased the tunnel down the length of my body, folding the spring downward until I was finally able to step out. Levi clapped as I hugged my hero.

With middle age, my shape transformed from a French fry to the whole potato.

This event probably would have never happened if it weren't for my ample waistline. My athletic, slender daughter would have shimmied out of that tunnel in seconds. And twenty years ago, I would have, too. With middle age, my shape transformed from a French fry to the whole potato. I fought against this shift at first. But trying different exercises and diets didn't work for me. Worrying about my clothing size was making me unhappy. Life is too short to be sad!

One day when Levi was an infant, I sat in the rocking chair with him. He was snuggled up and sound asleep, his body resting cozily on my stomach. "I guess you like my mattress," I whispered, stroking his hair. My attitude began to change a bit toward my "curves."

As Levi grew, I adored playing with him. I learned which slides at the park I fit on, and we "whooshed" down together. I could fit through the door of his playhouse, and accepted each invitation inside.

I learned which little chairs I could sit on without snapping them to bits like Goldilocks.

I was a large playmate, but I was always eager and available. Together, Levi and I make memories. I want him to remember his Grandma as a happy, smiling friend.

I may be a sphere instead of a cylinder, but there's more room for joy inside me. I'm as soft as a teddy bear and enjoy many loving squeezes. We share plenty of adventures and I hope he remembers each one, even the day I got 'tuck!

~Marianne Fosnow

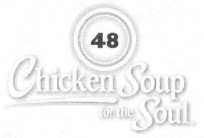

48

Living Big and Beautiful

*Sex appeal is fifty percent what you've got and fifty
percent what people think you've got.*
~Sophia Loren

I have never been skinny. Much to my chagrin, I don't believe I ever will be. I have calves too big for knee-high boots, thighs that rub together, arms that jiggle, and a chin with a twin. For many years I believed these were flaws and wondered if I could be loved.

No one believes me, but I am healthy. Really healthy. I get sick about once every five years, and it only lasts for about three days. I am strong as an ox and have stronger legs than a cross-country runner. I can lift 45 pounds with one arm. I can walk five miles straight without stopping. My blood pressure is low, as are my sugars. I am healthy.

After struggling with my self-image for many years, I made the decision that I would accept myself exactly as I was. Despite deciding this, I struggled with these things. Deciding is one thing, practicing is another. I have plenty to love and appreciate about myself. I am independent, smart, funny, caring, and creative, but I am "fat."

Try as I did, it took seeing myself through other people's eyes to finally appreciate myself physically. I had always received compliments on my looks, but dismissed them. Friends and family would rave about how beautiful I was. One day I met a wonderful man, who has forced me to see myself as he does, and finally accept how others see me.

He is teaching me that I am beautiful exactly as I am. He tells me how beautiful those things I thought of as flaws are. He shows me his appreciation of who I am inside and out, with constant reminders of his love. I have learned to accept those things I saw as flaws and love my whole self. I appreciate who I am and present myself with an air of confidence and comfort.

> *After struggling with my self-image for many years, I made the decision that I would accept myself exactly as I was.*

This is what I have needed. This is what I have been waiting for. I have never needed to be prettier, thinner, smarter, funnier. I have only needed to be me. Beautiful, unique me. We are all perfectly ourselves. This world needs us exactly as we are. Always work toward a better you, but never wish you were better. You are just what you are supposed to be.

~Danielle Sibila

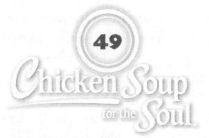

49

Kick, One, Two, Three...

The most terrifying thing is to accept
oneself completely.
~Carl Gustav Jung

The dance floor was empty. My group was up next. I took a deep breath and stepped into place with my fellow dancers. The better dancers stood in the front, but I didn't care. I knew what I could do. The music started and I moved across the floor with confidence and grace. I understood the purpose of the dance and I showed the emotion on my face and let my body do the rest. As I took the last step, I held my arms beautifully curved at my sides, slightly in front of my belly. I'd done well.

I took my seat on the side of the stage and waited for the rest of the groups to finish their final routines. The dance instructor looked gruff as he made his way to the stage. He walked by all of us, with pompous disinterest, and then reversed his path and started to point out individuals.

"You. You. You. Jerry. Sue..." He went on. "If I just pointed to you... you can leave the stage. Thank you. Maybe I'll see you at the next auditions."

I was a little surprised that I was still on stage.

"The rest of you... we'll see you here Monday night at 6:30 P.M."
With that, I was cast in *Can-Can*, my forty-eighth show and

thirty-ninth musical. For twenty-plus years, I've been a fat, funny, confident, character actress, paid singer and reluctant dancer. I wasn't like other entertainers, I was *me*. I had a thick waist, flabby arms and a round face, but I was talented and that trumped all the negatives that society might throw at me.

On Monday as I sat in the theater waiting for the rest of the cast, staff, and directors to arrive I realized that the stage was my life. It was the one place where I thrived and was accepted for who I was. I was comfortable here; my talent could shine.

After the director arrived, his assistant handed out scripts and I discovered I was a chorus member, background dancer and bit character. Fine with me. That meant I was going to be seen throughout the entire show. Nice!

A week into rehearsals, we were working on two of the longer dances and I realized the director was following my every move. Fifteen minutes later, the director called the dance instructor over to talk. They both turned to look at me, they talked a little more and then I was called over. My heart stuck in my throat. Was I being released from the show?

"Candace, right?" the director said.

"Yes," I said quietly.

"I hired you because I thought you'd be funny doing the can-can."

He smiled. "What I didn't expect is that you can actually dance." He patted the instructor on the shoulder. "Davis is going to re-stage the dances and you're going to be showcased. I have no doubt you can handle a full-fledged character dance." He turned to Davis. "Have her ready by next Tuesday."

For the next four days, I rehearsed and re-rehearsed the new steps. By Tuesday, I was ready. The music started and I was good and funny. All eyes were on me. The curvy girl showing all my fellow thespians that we have a place in this world.

Opening night was an explosion of emotions. I recalled all the staging, remembered all the lines and did all the dance steps perfectly. What I remembered most was the laughter. Guffaws for a comedic actor are the breaths of life, they're what keep us going and make us want to do it again and again and again. I couldn't wait to do it again the next day.

When I woke late the next morning, I checked the entertainment page in my newspaper to read about our opening night. As expected, the leads all got high scores and kudos. What stopped my heart was the write-up that I'd received. My name was pulled out of the cast and the critic gave me my own review.

> *Quirky, funny and she can dance. Candace Carteen adds charm and laughter to an almost perfect evening performance. A tried and true entertainer, she understands her character and puts all her weight behind it. No pun intended.*

Over and over again I scanned the words. I'd been honored before, but this particular writer had been less than kind to me in the past. Something had changed in both of us. Maybe it was the fact that I didn't care what others thought anymore. Maybe it was because the critic now had a little girl that was chunky. Whatever the reason, we weren't the people we were a few years ago.

After so many years of being bullied to be someone I wasn't, I decided that being me was a great thing.

I think that's true for anyone who is different and not perfect by society's standards. I'd been bullied my whole life, starting in childhood. My own father refused to teach me how to golf because my boobs were too big. After so many years of being bullied to be someone I wasn't, I decided that being me was a great thing.

If you ask my friends to describe me, they'd say I am empathic, caring, sweet, adaptable, loving, smart, charming, dedicated, financially in-tune and a great listener. That's not bad. They'd also add stubborn, tactless, and bitchy once in a while.

Being who I am has made me who I am. Does that mean that I no longer hear the ugly words that sad people sometimes throw at me on the street? No. Does it mean that I'm able to forgive all of those who have hurt me in the past? No.

It means that now I can say to myself, "What others think of me is none of my business."

That's powerful. After years of self-loathing, I've learned that I'm the person *I* have to live with every day. All I can do is be the best me I can.

I'm never going to be Twiggy. I wouldn't want to be. I want to be me. Curvy, funny, charismatic *me*! If you don't like that... I don't really care.

~Candace Carteen

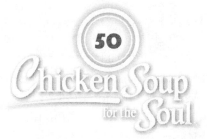

50

Two Bathing Suits

It's hard to fight an enemy who has
outposts in your head.
~Sally Kempton

I had always struggled with body issues. I had a very difficult childhood, and I was taught to be ashamed of myself. If I gained weight, I was scrutinized. If I lost weight, I was questioned, too.

I learned to make myself disappear to avoid getting in trouble. That meant not eating, or trying to snack on something late at night when everyone was asleep.

Once I got married, I had a supportive husband and I started eating better. I wasn't overweight by any measure, but I still felt shame about my body.

The only time I ever felt good about myself was when I was pregnant. I knew my body was performing an incredibly important role, the nurturing of life. I realized how much strength and power I had as a woman, a mother.

Of course, postpartum, all of those feelings quickly disappeared.

The yo-yo diets started again, and it was always the same thing: Lose and feel great. Gain and feel like a complete failure.

Some years ago, I lost all of the excess weight. I felt amazing, on top of the world! I couldn't believe I actually did it. Shopping was suddenly so much fun, as opposed to the dread I used to feel in those horribly lit fitting rooms. I had such confidence; I thought nothing could get in my way.

Until I put the weight back on, and then some.

Last year we were planning a trip to Greece. That meant beautiful beaches and plenty of time in bathing suits. I was excited and horrified at the same time. What was I going to do? I knew deep down that I would regret hiding myself. If I didn't get in the water with my family I would feel terrible.

When the time came to shop for a bathing suit, I was terrified. My eleven-year-old son offered to go with me for support.

> *I walked out of the store with two bathing suits that day, a first for me.*

When I found one that seemed to fit, even though I hated how I looked, I let my son come into the changing room to see it. His eyes grew wide and he said, "Mama, you look so beautiful!"

I started to tear up then and there, and he hugged me, repeating himself, and asked me to please buy not only the one I was wearing, but the other one in another color as well.

I walked out of the store with two bathing suits that day, a first for me.

That summer, I spent as much time as possible in the sea, and it was the most incredible, healing experience I had had in a long time. When we went for a boat tour in the Aegean, we had the opportunity to go snorkeling. My son took my hand and we went into the water together.

This summer, I am looking forward to pools and beaches yet again. My body shame has disappeared, and I have never felt better about myself.

My son had no idea what he did for me, but it was transformative, and I am so grateful to him.

~Tamara Albanna

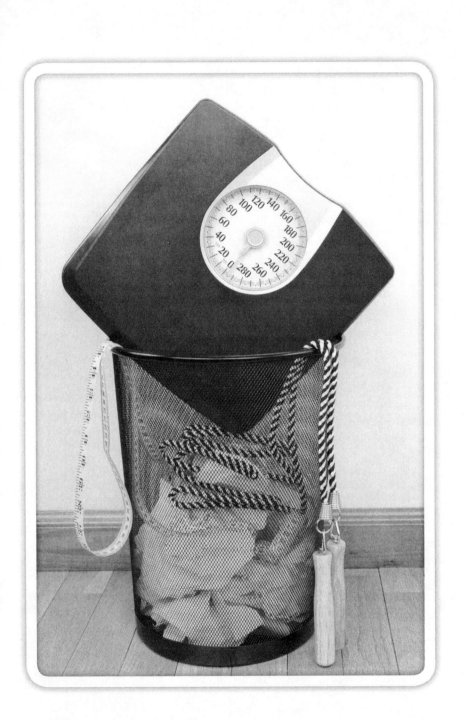

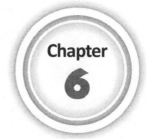

Chapter
6

Curvy & Confident

Warning, Dangerous Curves

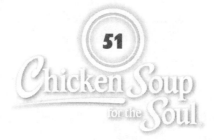

51

The Green Dress

Confidence is the sexiest thing a woman can have. It's
much sexier than any body part.
~Aimee Mullins

My daughter Rina called. "Mom, everyone in the wedding party is wearing green. I expect you to as well."

"Baby, I was planning to wear my black dress."

"No. I want you to look pretty."

I gave myself a pep talk. *The bride's always right. Brides should have the wedding of their dreams. She's getting married in three months so maybe I can get into shape?*

I sat on my bed, avoiding the mirror. It would reflect a tall woman with curly hair and glasses, wearing a sloppy gray sweat suit.

Oh, yes, and 30 extra pounds. It had been a long time since I'd felt pretty.

My fashion-conscious husband Larry, who'd wear a suit to the grocery store, dragged me shopping. But two months of retail hell later I still didn't have a dress.

Then, one day, I found it.

I came out of the dressing room and my husband's jaw dropped. The saleslady clapped. The jade green dress was long-sleeved and feminine. An attached duster floated around my body.

Touching the gold necklace sewn on the neckline, I was stunned. Was that woman in the mirror *me*? I hadn't worn a clingy dress like this in years. My husband and the saleslady even made me change into a smaller size to show off my curves!

Larry kissed my hand, then twirled me around. "You look so fine. I can hardly wait to show you off."

When I looked at my reflection, I didn't see flaws. The green dress celebrated my curvy figure.

> *Why had I hidden my curvy body in dull colors and loose styles all those years? Being* me *was wonderful!*

A month later, I cried when Rina glided down the aisle in her fairy princess gown, a green-eyed beauty with jade ribbons swaying from her bouquet.

My appearance shocked friends and family. Why had I hidden my curvy body in dull colors and loose styles all those years? Being *me* was wonderful! In between dances at the reception, a stranger approached me. Beautiful, toned, and curvy, she looked at me enviously. "Where did you get that spectacular dress? You look beautiful."

The lesson I learned from that green dress is simple: Love yourself, love your curves. You're beautiful.

~Karla Brown

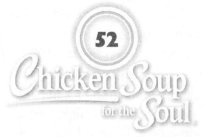
Perfectly Imperfect

No one can make you feel inferior
without your consent.
~Eleanor Roosevelt

n the last day of fifth grade, a boy in my class was reciting the alphabet out loud and matching each letter with the name of a classmate in the room. "A is for Anna, B is for Brian… " When he reached the letter "E" he looked around but couldn't find a student with an "E" name, so he pointed at me: "Elephant!" My classmates snickered.

It was just one of many bullying incidents I'd experienced at school because of my weight. After school that day, I walked home in tears. But deep within the pain and anger, a strength rose from within me. I swore to myself that from that moment on, my life would change. I would never again let anyone diminish me by calling me names and I would never let my weight stop me from doing anything I wanted to do.

The following year, in sixth grade, I began using humor as a tool to win the approval and admiration of my peers. Instead of hiding behind my weight, I put myself out there in full force. And I discovered something wonderful: I liked myself. That revelation amazed me and I no longer felt like a victim. Now I was in charge of how people treated me. I fast became one of the most popular kids in school and maintained that status throughout my school years by utilizing humor and kindness. My senior year I was a plus-sized Homecoming Queen. I felt as rare as a unicorn.

After graduating from the University of Michigan I headed to New York City to pursue my dream to be a plus-size model, landing a contract with Ford Models. It was the late 1980's and I was one of the pioneers of the plus-size industry, along with my dear friend Emme. In a sea of muumuus and polyester pull-on pants, being a plus model was being an advocate for women's empowerment.

But while I felt sexy and curvy, I was often made to look older and without sensuality in my photos. The photographers (at the command of the clients) told the plus models to "smile at the camera." The subtext was: You're a plus talent so be a one-dimensional, fat and happy figurine. The blatant prejudicial treatment was everywhere we turned in an industry that valued a specific type of physical perfection above all.

> *I headed to New York City to pursue my dream to be a plus-size model, landing a contract with Ford Models.*

When I shot spreads for a leading department store, they had us do our own hair and make-up before arriving on set. Our shoots were scheduled early in the morning and by having me arrive "shoot-ready," they could finish quickly before shooting "straight-size" models — as in, *real* models. As I was in front of the camera shooting my outfits, I'd watch as the thin models had their hair and make-up done by a professional. In the client's eyes, plus models were not even worthy of hiring a make-up artist. The unmistakable message: You're not beautiful; you're only necessary for us to make sales to second-class citizens.

I tried not to let the painful message diminish me. But there were times I could feel the old shame bubble up from within, scars from my childhood, and I would wonder if I deserved any of what I had worked so hard to create. How could I be a model in New York City, signed with the greatest agency in the world? I have cellulite. I have rolls. I weigh over 200 pounds, and I am full of imperfections. At those times, I wanted nothing more than to dive into a half gallon of ice cream in a vicious cycle of self-punishment.

It was on a day such as this that I was lying on my chiropractor's table staring at the ceiling, feeling fat, ugly, lost and alone.

I've always had a strong faith, so I started to talk to God. I prayed that He would heal the pain and shame inside me. Then, a flash of clarity washed over me as I realized: "You are perfectly imperfect."

When I looked up, I saw a beautiful woman with long blond hair and a diaphanous white gown floating above me, surrounded by a glowing white light. She was smiling at me, laughing lovingly with a twinkle in her eyes as if to say, "Of course you are, silly!" Then she kissed my cheek and faded away. I was in shock and in tears, wondering if I had just hallucinated, dreamed it, or if someone had slipped me a drug. The air in the room felt like it had shifted.

A moment later, my doctor walked in and stopped dead in his tracks, asking, "What just happened in here?" He felt it. It had really happened. He confirmed it without seeing anything.

Was my vision an angel, my guardian, or my higher-self whispering a reminder of my own deepest wisdom? It doesn't even matter; she was a miracle to me.

Since that life-changing day, I've had days when I've struggled with self-acceptance, but I've never doubted that I am supported and loved, and never alone.

My "angel" reminded me of what I already knew: I am perfectly imperfect, worthy of love and the realization of my dreams. And so are you, my friend. So are you.

~Alexandra Boos

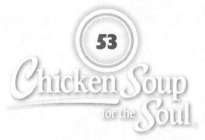

53

Baby Got Back to Basics

Your chances of success in any undertaking can always
be measured by your belief in yourself.
~Robert Collier

When I was a young theater student in college, I auditioned for a production of a one-act play about dating in the modern world. I got the part of a sarcastic, bookish woman at a bar who shoots down a man's cheesy pick-up lines and throws a glass of water in his face.

It was great fun, but the most interesting part was how the director wanted us to bow at the end. He wanted us to do something unique. On a dare, the cast decided it would be a grand idea to arrive onstage at the end of the play wearing only our underwear and dance to Sir Mix-a-Lot's "Baby Got Back," the ultimate ode to curvy women.

Just shy of 5'9" with measurements of 36-27-36 — I had a near perfect hourglass figure, taller and built more solidly than most women. My legs looked great too, and I had a pretty face. I was a "knockout" by traditional beauty standards, but I didn't know it.

I thought my body was too large to be shown in public. I wanted to hide it.

Opening night approached for the play. Everyone was readying their costumes, perfecting their lines, and memorizing the choreography for the final bow sequence. I figured it was only two nights of my life, and the underwear set I'd chosen was more modest than many a swimsuit I'd worn, so not too much harm could be done.

The play went off without a hitch. The audience laughed uproariously when I threw the glass of water in my suitor's face, and at the end, I stood tallest in the center of the dance line, in my underwear, waiting for the final curtain. I breathed deeply and reassured myself that this moment could not kill me; I would survive it, even if I had to pick rotten tomatoes out of my hair afterward.

As the rap song played and we danced in unison, the audience rolled with laughter. It was an unexpected celebration of comedy and confidence in a world of dating disasters. We'd won the night, and I'd kept my promise to my director and myself.

> *I stood tallest in the center of the dance line, in my underwear, waiting for the final curtain.*

After the show, the cast dressed and waited in the lobby to meet the audience. I was unprepared for the flood of emotions that followed. We'd just put on a light-hearted comedy about finding love in a crazy world, and as audience members came to greet me, one by one, they shook my hand or hugged me tight. Not so much for my performance, but for my bravery to go onstage in my underwear.

Women of all sizes couldn't wait to tell me how my costume choice had emboldened them to be themselves. In tears, some told me they were going to go home and pull out the lingerie or bathing suit they never wore or had stuffed in the back of their closet, explaining that they now felt beautiful enough to put them on.

I'd simply kept my word on a dare, in the name of comedy — and somehow, I'd brought these women love of their own beauty. There is no better reward in acting than to empower the members of your audience to go forth and love themselves.

Especially when it takes you by surprise because you were simply being your vulnerable, imperfect self.

~A. Kay Wyatt

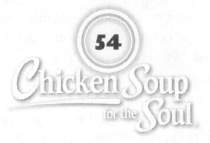

54

Cracked Rear View

Embrace your curves and who you are. I feel proud if
young girls look up to me and say, "I'm curvy,
and I'm proud of it now."
~Kim Kardashian

It happened in the shower. There I was, soap in hand, minding my own business, when I thought, *You know, having a curvy butt really isn't a bad thing.* This was a huge improvement for me. Normally, I'd look in the mirror and I'd think, *Good lord, why does my butt have to look like a shelf?*

For a white girl, I have a lot of booty. Whether that's a blessing or a curse depends on your point of view. Viewed by my husband, it is a blessing. However, until my recent revelation, I viewed my posterior as a very large and inconvenient curse.

Until I was about twelve, I had a pretty normal girl's body. I was fairly lean, long legged, the tallest in my sixth grade class. But once puberty hit — bam! Up jumped the booty. The older I got, the more it kept jumping.

Clothes that fit were harder to find. In the late 1970's, wearing boys Levi's jeans was all the rage. But boys Levi's weren't cut to accommodate a Rubenesque behind. Actually, no pants were. If they fit my bum, I had to tie up the waist like a burlap sack. Not a great look.

I learned to make do. That's code for "I wore a lot of skirts." My parents let me dress to the nines for school, even in junior high. If nothing else, I was fashionable. Still, I didn't feel very attractive. I had one boyfriend in high school who liked me just the way I was. But I was too stupid and insecure to believe him, so he gave up on me. I can't say that I blame him.

My rear view stayed pretty much the same through college and my twenties. At thirty, I was newly married and very much in love with a man who admired my shape. Fashion had changed, was more accommodating of my least favorite asset. But neither of these improved my attitude about my overly generous genetic jackpot.

A few years later, a series of family tragedies, combined with lengthy and expensive fertility treatments, gave my system a one-two punch. I was a stress eater and a worrier. My cortisol was through the roof and so was my caloric intake. I gained a lot of weight. Guess where most of it went?

I started wondering if my problem was not in my bum, but in my head.

As I ventured through two pregnancies, postpartum depression, and the hormonal imbalances that accompany aging (thank you *so* much, Mother Nature), the rumpus just kept growing.

Some days I felt like my bum deserved its own zip code. But, no one else seemed to notice. No one pointed as I walked down the street. I started wondering if my problem was not in my bum, but in my head.

A few years ago, I decided to make some changes. I took better charge of my physical and mental health. I dropped some weight and got my system back in balance. My rear view got a little smaller. Not a lot, but enough to make me feel better.

Then I noticed the world had changed again.

Stores sold expensive shapewear promising to make women's bums look full and curvy. Female entertainers had ample posteriors that earned them lots of appreciation and big bucks. Women were paying plastic surgeons thousands of dollars for something called a Brazilian butt lift.

I looked in the mirror and thought: *Wow, what am I complaining about? I have all this... for free!*

Finally, I started believing my husband's compliments (and the glimmer in his eye). I started thinking that just maybe I wasn't the unlucky one, that maybe the real problem had been in my head all along, and not in my rear end. And, to paraphrase the great philosopher Pumba (the fat funny one in *The Lion King*), I started putting my attitude about my behind in my past.

And this morning, after all this time, I found acceptance in the shower. Who would've thunk it.

So what if I'll never fit into boys Levi's or model haute couture. I like who I am. At forty-eight, I can rock a fitted skirt and 4" heels like nobody's business while juggling a successful career, setting a healthy example for my growing daughter, and inspiring lust in the man I love every day of every week.

There isn't a skinny jean model in the world I would trade places with now.

~Cindi Carver-Futch

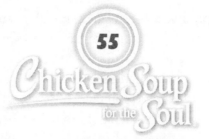

55

For the Love of Curves

It is confidence in our bodies, minds, and spirits that
allows us to keep looking for new adventures.
~Oprah Winfrey

I ran into the house gasping for breath, with tears running down my cheeks, and my chest heaving. I was nearly hyperventilating. Between sobs I managed to tell my alarmed mom, "I'm so ugly."

Some kids at my after-school program, a few I called friends, decided to give me a nickname — "Garfield," — you know, after the orange, fat, lazy cat. As you can imagine, this is not how a seven-year-old girl wants to be identified. Whether I got the name because I had big expressive, sleepy eyes or because I was a plump kid, I knew with every fiber of my seven-year-old self that I was ugly, because that's what everyone said, so it must be true.

My mother hugged me, wiped my tears, and told me I was beautiful.

"Crying just hides the beauty, so don't cry and don't listen to those kids. Listen to me and listen to what you know about yourself. You're beautiful and smart. No one's words can change that."

From that point on, the words "I'm ugly" were banished from my vocabulary, replaced with "I'm beautiful, I'm confident." My mom provided the foundation for my confidence, and because of that, I'm now a plus-size model and body positive blogger who helps other curvy women find their confidence.

I coined the phrase #ForTheLoveOfCurves and explore body

confidence and positive self-esteem on my blog, curvygirlchronicles.net, where I share stories of body acceptance and self-love and spotlight inspirational female entrepreneurs working in the plus-size industry or who have a body positive message.

People ask how I learned to embrace my curves. I recently developed a fun challenge to help other women embrace their bodies. I call it the Body Image Detox.

> *My mom provided the foundation for my confidence.*

On social media, you can find so many advertisements for detox teas or cleanses to get our bodies right. But what about getting our minds in the right place about our bodies? When I need to undo the damage from media images that say things like only flat stomachs are beautiful, I go to my detox.

The body image detox has seven steps ranging from actively posting a video on social media about how I embrace my body, to posting positive quotes about body image. I know I'm reaching others and spreading Mom's message of confidence when I get responses like: "I love the body message that you are sending to new generations. Making every single type of body feel beautiful. Empowering every woman to feel pretty, strong and self-sufficient."

Wow! Seven-year-old me would be proud; I do this for her, for my future children, for the women who read my blog, and for the love of curves.

Take that, Garfield!

~Kristina Bigby

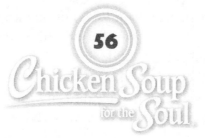

56

Three B

*The only person who can pull me down is myself, and
I'm not going to let myself pull me down anymore.*
~C. JoyBell C.

Mama frowned and shook her head. "Just look at those feet. Wouldn't they look odd hanging at the end of a pair of skinny legs?"

At age twelve, I already wore size 8 shoes. I was on the verge of tears, despondent about being the largest girl in my class. While the boys at school were starting to notice the slim, pretty girls, the only attention I got from them was when they teased me about my size.

I glowered at Mama. "You don't understand because you've never been fat."

Mama gave me a hug. "You aren't fat, Betty. You're just a big girl. You have to learn to love your sturdy, strong body. We all have to take what we're given in life and make the most of it."

She stroked my hair. "People usually think of you exactly as you think of yourself. If you continue to go around with your head down and your shoulders slumped you're telling the world that you aren't much. But if you stand tall, walk proud, and smile they will see something in you that makes them want to know you."

Desperate, I tried Mama's advice. I joined in the games at recess, laughed and pretended to be confident. I learned that if I joked and horsed around, kids were drawn to me. Slowly, I made friends and became one of the popular kids. I was now known as the big girl with the great personality. But it was all a farce. Everything on the outside was a charade while on the inside, I still felt insecure… and fat.

Every year I got taller and bigger while most of the other pudgy girls slimmed down. If I voiced my disdain at my body, I'd hear: "But you are so well proportioned. You have such nice curves. You're not fat, you're just large."

Still, nothing they said could make me think I was anything but gawky and fat.

I didn't date in high school. Teenage boys don't go for big girls. Mama assured me that the boys in college were more mature and would appreciate my own brand of beauty. Mama was wrong. Oh, the guys thought I was great, hilarious and always ready for a good time.

> *"Three B is his pet name for you: Big, Beautiful Betty."*

But when it came to romance they reached for the smaller girls.

During my last year in college I was late getting to a party. When I pushed through the throng of dancing kids, trying to find my friends, I heard a loud voice call out: "Where is Three B?"

I wondered whom he was referring to when I noticed several heads swivel toward me. "Here she is," someone said. I forced myself to grin even though my heart fell with a devastated thud. What did Three B mean? Were they making fun me?

I spotted my best friend, Jane, and hurried over to her.

"What does Three B mean?" I asked, whispering.

Jane looked at my pinched face and laughed. "Relax. That is what Joe always calls you. He is crazy about you but hasn't gotten up the nerve to ask you out. Three B is his pet name for you: Big, Beautiful Betty. Get it? Three B's."

Joe approached, blushing and grinning. "You weren't supposed to hear that, but now that you have, it's the only thing I will ever call you. Want to dance, Three B?"

Joe and I married after college and true to his word he has never called me anything else.

Through the years since then, I still dreamed of slimming down. I tried dieting and lost weight, but got haggard and tired looking. With every pound I lost, I seemed to lose a bit of spark. I felt better when I was what Mama always said was my natural size. So, for a long time I stopped trying to lose weight. I wasn't happy with my size but I hid my feelings behind my bubbly personality and laughter.

Then, my niece, Angie, asked me to be the matron of honor in her wedding.

I stood in front of my full-length mirror and cringed at the thought of wedding pictures. *I'll dwarf everyone else. She'll regret asking me to be in her wedding.*

For the first time in years I dieted again. I measured every mouthful of food I ate and walked every evening after dinner. I grew tired and cranky but I was determined to lose weight before the wedding.

During spring break at college, Angie came to visit and show me pictures of the dresses she had chosen for her bridesmaids and me. Her eyes filled with concern when I opened the door. "Aunt Betty, are you sick?" Her eyes scanned my body. "What's wrong? You've lost weight."

I laughed and led her to the kitchen so we could chat and she could eat the brownies I'd baked for her.

"I'm fine, honey. I've been dieting so I'll look better for your wedding."

She frowned. "Well, it isn't working. You look awful."

"But you don't want an elephant to stand beside you at your wedding," I said, trying to laugh. But the sound was forced and hollow as I looked at her disappointed face.

She crossed her arms and gave me a steady gaze.

"Aunt Betty, when I thought my nose was too big, you told me that when I got older and my face finished taking shape, my nose would look just fine. Then, when I fussed about my curly hair and wanted to straighten it, you told me to work with what I had because natural was better. And when I hated being short and tiny, you assured me that many men love petite girls."

Her eyes narrowed. "I believed every word you said because you always accepted yourself and worked with what you had. But you must not believe it yourself, because here you are trying to mold yourself into something you're not."

Tears sprang into her eyes. "I asked Three B to be my matron of honor and she is who I want to stand with me. Did you forget what the name means? I was always proud of Big, Beautiful Betty. My friends at college can't wait to meet her. But," she shook her head, "you're becoming a nervous, washed-out, sick-looking shell of her."

I grabbed the brownie from Angie's plate and took a bite. Angie looked shocked for a moment, then laughed.

"I love you just the way you are," she said, giving me a hug. "Everyone does."

"I will, too." I said with conviction. "From this moment on I will."

And I have.

~Elizabeth Atwater

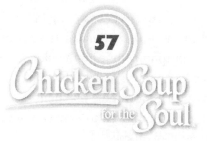

57

Beauty at Every Size

The beauty of a woman must be seen from in her
eyes, because that is the doorway to her heart, the
place where love resides.
~Audrey Hepburn

Feeling beautiful has always been very important to me. Yet through all the years that I hated my body, it didn't matter what size I was, a part of me wasn't willing to consider myself beautiful. The truth was I never saw a full-figured woman whose face showed confidence that she felt beautiful exactly as she was.

In early 2009, in the process of writing my book, *Lovin' the Skin You're In*, I stumbled upon a plus-size model magazine website. I was overjoyed to discover a whole other world of beauty. I scrolled through the online magazine and read article after article about fashion, movies, events, and many other wonderful things. It opened up my world, expanded my vision, increased my appreciation for my body, and made me feel beautiful inside and out.

I clicked through the pages and saw a sisterhood of beautiful women of all sizes and shapes. Suddenly, I didn't feel like an outcast. Seeing my body through fresh eyes made my confidence soar. And that felt so good that I just had to spread the love and inspire other women to see their bodies as beautiful, too.

One day I was shopping in Lane Bryant for summer blouses. I buzzed through the store making my choices from the racks and plucking out an armload of clothes ranging in size from 14/16–18/20.

As I headed to the fitting room to try my clothes on, a lovely woman stopped to compliment me on the blouse I was wearing. It was a short-sleeved peasant blouse with a blue and green mosaic design.

When I dressed that morning, I had deliberately pulled down the elasticized neckline of the blouse to expose my neck and shoulders because I loved that look on me.

As I glanced at the woman who complimented my blouse, I noticed her eyes had a wistful expression. I wondered why. Then I smiled at her and said, "You know this same blouse would look incredible on you." I pointed to the rack and told her, "I bought it here. It's still available. What do you think of getting it?"

Suddenly, I didn't feel like an outcast.

I watched as her lovely smile faded and the corners of her mouth turned down. She said, "Oh no, my arms are too fat. That type of blouse is not for me."

I told her that those negative thoughts were probably coming from the screaming meanie critics inside her head, the ones that were holding her back from wearing these pretty blouses and doing the other things she really wanted to do.

I explained a little further about how we all have an internal voice that can make us doubt ourselves, that tells us to be afraid and believe we're not good enough or pretty enough. Then I reminded her that she's the one in charge, not that voice, and she could take back control anytime she wanted.

I had been through the same things myself. So many years lost to self-doubt. For years, I wouldn't have had the confidence to bare my arms in public no matter what size I was. Reading that online magazine had changed things for me. I was tired of hating myself and feeling ashamed of my appearance. I was finally ready to accept myself as I was, with all my imperfections intact. No more sitting around and waiting for perfect. Not me.

Later as I stood at the counter paying for my purchases, I noticed the woman was also there. I asked if she bought the blouse. She shook her head and said, "No, I didn't, but I got a very similar one. You inspired me. I feel better about myself now."

I count that as a triumph over the meanies. My guess is that this lovely woman finally got a glimpse of herself through someone else's eyes, in this case, mine. In the same way that seeing curvy women model beautiful clothes in a magazine inspired me to see myself as beautiful, this woman was inspired by seeing me. Just for a moment, she stepped outside the boundaries she had made for herself and saw what was possible.

~Andrea Amador

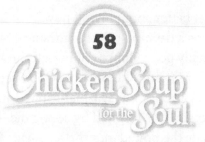

58

Perfect Fit

*Once you accept the fact that you're not perfect, then
you develop some confidence.*
~Rosalynn Carter

What a happy day. I'm doing a happy dance, because I have found jeans that fit. Yes, they're curvy-fit jeans that stretch a little to fit. Thanks to 2% Spandex added to the denim, I sized down to one size smaller than I usually wear. There are those that call this vanity sizing, but in my mind, it's a confidence booster. I now own these jeans in three colors: black, white and blue denim.

Growing up, I was often teased about my size. I was too tall, too fat, too different. My mom's words of encouragement still linger with me: "It's the size of your heart that matters, not the size of your clothes." I have tried to live my life by that philosophy, but it hasn't been easy.

I was ten years old when I experienced my first sleepless night and tear-stained pillow from agonizing over the realization that I was different.

It happened during Christmas break. My best friend and I were playing a game in my bedroom, while our mothers were in the kitchen having coffee and sharing sewing tips, ideas, patterns, and fabrics. "I know it's easier for me to make a skirt for my petite daughter, but here's a skirt pattern I think our daughters will love," my friend's mother said. "Look at this lovely soft, navy blue wool remnant I bought on sale. Since your daughter is taller and big-boned, do you think there's enough fabric to make each girl a skirt?"

"Adjusting a pattern for my beautiful daughter isn't difficult," Mom replied. "All I have to do is add an inch or two here and there. There's definitely enough material to make them matching skirts."

After hearing every hurtful word, my eyes welled with tears, as I surmised being tall, big-boned and beautiful wasn't a good thing.

"Don't cry," my friend said, "I don't think you're fat."

From that day forward, I was grateful for my mom's support as I struggled to fit in as the tall, big-boned girl with the pretty face. All through school, Mom was my champion. She insisted I ignore those who taunted me about my size. Eventually, I learned to do that, which helped build my confidence to participate in many school activities. I became an editor of the school newspaper, joined the glee club, performed in several school plays, and got good grades. Granted, I was still the tall, big-boned girl with the pretty face, but I no longer dwelled on my image in the mirror every day.

> *I'm doing a happy dance, because I have found jeans that fit.*

Once I left the nest and was launched into adulthood, I chose a career in the corporate world of financial management. However, during the interview process, there were five other applicants seated with me in the front lobby. We were all seeking the same position. I wanted to get up and leave… all five applicants were attractive, petite women. How could I possibly be considered for the job? Suddenly, a sense of shame washed over me for having such negative thoughts. Quickly, I pushed them aside and one of Mom's pep talks came to mind, "Take a deep breath. You're smart, you've got this."

Because of that nudge to bolster my self-esteem, I aced the interview. Not only did I land the job, but six months later I met my husband-to-be, who always preferred tall, big-boned, beautiful and confident women.

Today I modeled my new black jeans for my husband and he whistled softly, "Wow, those are a great pair of jeans."

"They're the new curvy-fit style," I said as I performed an exaggerated runway strut.

My husband smiled. "There's nothing wrong with being curvy,

and I like curves."

I love that man of mine for loving and accepting me for who I am. We've just celebrated thirty-eight years of wedded bliss. Indeed, we're the perfect fit.

Even though many years have passed, my mom's words of wisdom are still relevant today, "It's the size of your heart that matters, not the size of your clothes."

~Georgia A. Hubley

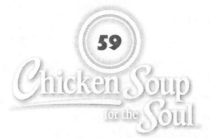

59

The Curves Within

Believing in our hearts that who we are is enough is the
key to a more satisfying and balanced life.
~Ellen Sue Stern

I slowly closed the laptop and fixed my stare on a distant corner of the living room. What was wrong with me? How did I cause this?

I'd just finished reading my spouse's Facebook messages in which she proclaimed her love to a co-worker, a woman I didn't know.

"Ten years," I thought. "We wasted ten years assembling a life, a home, and a family."

Why did this happen? *The cheater I married was at work, probably flirting and stoking the affair just as I was learning about it.*

My one-year-old sighed, asleep in her swing a few feet from where I sat. I looked down at my bulging thighs. I gained 60 pounds while pregnant, and though a year had passed since giving birth, I had not lost the weight.

It's me, I thought. *I let myself go.*

Before this moment, I was okay with my appearance. I had the hips and rump that ran in my family, but I was skilled at dressing my curves. "Good, childbearing hips," my five aunts always said, and they were right — my pregnancy and delivery went off without a hitch.

I thought I was handling the weight gain with grace, focusing on my daughter's needs. Now I realized I might not be as attractive as I had felt, especially to the person for whom it mattered most — my spouse. My confidence shattered.

The infidelity continued for a couple of months even after I confronted my spouse, chipping away at more of my self-esteem with every lie I uncovered. I kept the affair a secret from everyone we knew, choosing not to smear our reputations, telling myself I could bounce back from this on my own. But I couldn't.

I felt worthless, ashamed, and focused the blame and self-hate on my appearance. It wasn't just my curves I blamed. I hated my brown eyes and my olive-toned skin. I hated my knees and stopped wearing shorts. I internalized every wrong done to me and took apart my self-image, telling myself I wasn't as intelligent as I once believed, as funny, or as good a mother.

> *I felt worthless, ashamed, and focused the blame and self-hate on my appearance.*

My friends thought of me as a strong, independent woman who moved mountains to get what she wanted. I didn't feel like that woman anymore, and I began to believe that perhaps I never was.

One warm spring evening my best friend Robin asked if she could bring her kids by to play. She lived a few doors down, but we hadn't seen each other in months because I'd been avoiding everyone. I agreed, keeping my lips on lockdown during our visit and nodding from time to time as she updated me on her life since we last spoke. We sipped ice-cold water on the deck and watched the kids toddle in the yard.

"What is going on with you?" Robin finally asked, concerned.

I shook my head.

"You can tell me," she said.

I focused on the grass.

"You are not yourself. I've never seen you like this," she said.

The dam broke. All the emotions I carried — the self-loathing, the disappointment in my weight gain and appearance, the absolute hate of myself — spewed out of me. I unloaded each feeling and unpacked it before my friend.

News of the affair did not surprise her. How I allowed it to control my self-worth, however, shocked her. We talked through each of the things I thought was wrong with me, starting with my personality and eventually moving to my appearance. We spoke for hours.

My gorgeous friend, curvy and beautiful with a bright smile, brilliant mind and contagious laugh, showed me that I wasn't to blame for the affair, and neither was my appearance or my curves. She reminded me of all the times perfect strangers had hit on me because of my magnetic confidence.

Thankfully, my best friend's insight helped me begin to heal.

Since that day, with her support, I've been through divorce, therapy, and am now happily remarried and friends with my ex.

When I look in the mirror today, I once again see the strong, self-assured, brave, beautiful and curvy woman that I am.

~Mary Anglin-Coulter

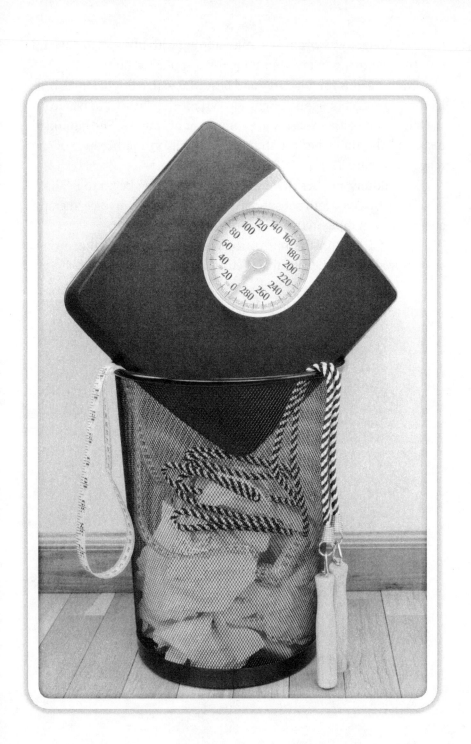

Curvy & Confident

The Joy of Exercise

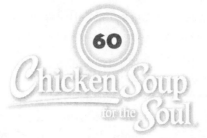

60

A Woman My Size

There are short-cuts to happiness, and
dancing is one of them.
~Vicki Baum

I walked into my first Zumba class with a nervous smile pasted on my face. About thirty women of all shapes and sizes — and a few brave men — stood in lines facing the stage. My black leggings and long, black T-shirt seemed dull next to their brightly colored outfits. Even the bigger women like me were wearing pink and yellow. What were they thinking?

Everyone was talking to each other, smiling, and hugging before the class began. As an overweight, reluctant exerciser, I was shocked by that. Being at the gym had never been a pleasant experience for me; I never sincerely grinned about exercising. I had always believed I was too fat to shake my butt in front of a roomful of strangers. Heck, I felt too fat to walk down the street because I'd been "mooed" at and called "whale" by people driving by.

A lean and fit woman dressed in neon and turquoise walked onstage and introduced herself as Lisa, the instructor. She turned on the music, turned off the lights, and a disco ball with dance lights spun around and lit up the room. People yelled and clapped like a concert was about to begin. Lisa started moving, pointing, and dancing. The class followed.

I couldn't do all the moves, like twisting my hips around in a circle, but before I knew it, I'd danced for an hour. My hair dripped with sweat and I was clapping along with everyone else. Yes, I clapped. I couldn't believe I'd exercised for that long without passing out. And it was fun! Wait, did I say that?

The magic of my first Zumba class motivated me to join the gym. I attended as many Zumba classes as I could, sometimes two a day. Every class made me feel better about moving my body.

The music, dancing, energy, fun, and magic of the classes made me feel free. I know that sounds corny, but it's true. The choreography challenged me to move in new ways and push myself physically, but it was never humiliating or painful, like other exercise programs I'd tried. For some reason, I didn't feel limited any more by my size or past battles with extra weight. I didn't feel trapped in a fat body anymore.

> *This weird, unexpected idea came into my head; I wanted to become a Zumba instructor.*

I was still overweight, but I wasn't self-conscious about my legs rubbing, my belly bouncing, or my need to wear two sports bras to feel comfortable while dancing around.

With the "fat limits" gone, something strange and unbelievable happened. This weird, unexpected idea came into my head; I wanted to become a Zumba instructor. I wanted to be a part of the group that helped bring so much joy to people like me.

Anyone who is motivated enough can become an instructor, I discovered. It's not about having six-pack abs or a rock-hard butt. It's about energy, enthusiasm, and motivating people to enjoy their own ability to move to music.

Still, when I arrived at my first Zumba Instructor class I panicked for a moment when I saw I wasn't as fit as most of the others. Then we all sat down and talked about why we wanted to become instructors. Many shared what I felt — that Zumba had saved them or someone they knew and they wanted to be a part of it. Some said that the dancing helped alleviate the sadness, self-hate, and hopelessness in their lives.

When we all got up to dance, I didn't care anymore that my butt was the biggest in the room. I shook it like everyone else.

Today, I'm a Zumba instructor and I love that I can help others have fun while exercising.

I'm not a size 2. I'm a size 14. I'm not cut like some instructors are and I still wear two sports bras. Yes, I've dropped some weight. But this is not a weight loss story; it's a freedom story. My butt is still big and I still jiggle, but I'm moving with pride. I stand in front of a group of people with a big smile on my face and when the music starts, I move and they move with me.

We dance. All sizes, all shapes, all ages.

I recently gave a Zumba demonstration at an event, and afterward an older man attempted to pay me a compliment: "For a woman your size, you move really well. You surprised me."

At one time, I might have been insulted, angry, or hurt by a comment like that. But now, I stood tall in my bright pink, extra-large exercise outfit.

"Go to Zumba and you'll never be surprised again."

With my big smile, big butt, and head held high... I left to go lead another routine.

~Darbie Andrews

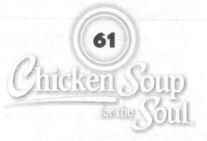
Slogging

*Your body will argue that there is no justifiable reason
to continue. Your only recourse is to call on your spirit,
which functions independently of logic.*
~Tim Noakes

I still remember those awful runs twenty years ago: four laps on a cinder track with the high school volleyball team in the hot Missouri summer. If anyone stopped running, we all had to start over. Afterwards, we lined up for lukewarm water, sweat dripping into our eyes, off our chins, and pooling around our shoes.

I didn't want to run again ever, until 2012, when everything changed. One friend of mine died and another became very ill with a degenerative disease. While overwhelmed with grief for them, I noticed that a lot of people I knew were starting to run. I couldn't conceive of a reason why anyone would take up such a hobby. The mere thought of it overwhelmed my memory with images of stern coaches, whistles at the ready, yelling to add another lap. I remembered the heat and the thirst, and the way my heart pounded and my lungs burned.

But you get to a point when you're out of shape and decide to either accept yourself the way you are or make a change. After nearly a decade of infertility, I'd given up on my body ever doing anything I wanted it to do.

Yet the death of my friend inspired me to make a change.

I saw my friends rejoicing in the stress relief and pride they got through running, beaming in photos at their 5K finish lines. They had something in common, something that appealed to me. They felt *alive* when they ran.

And in the shadow of my friends' death and illness, I wanted to feel alive, too. Not just for me, but for them. When I remembered my teenage disdain for running and the burning lungs and aching legs, it occurred to me that every single day, people die too young all over this planet. Wouldn't they give anything to have one more day to walk on this earth, let alone run?

And so, with more than 60 pounds to lose, I strapped on a new pair of running shoes, downloaded a training app, and wondered if I should warn my neighbors: "Hey, gang, if you see something disturbing prowling the streets, it's just me. I'm becoming a runner."

With my friends on my mind, I started up the hill in front of our house.

After twelve years of infertility, I was pregnant.

It had to be a hill.

I don't know if you could call what I was doing "running." I called it a "sloppy jog" for so long that I began to refer to my runs as "going slogging."

Each time I went slogging instead of sleeping or eating or shopping, I was taking back control of my body. Soon, I was managing longer runs. A six-mile workout was not uncommon on the weekends.

Finally, in the fall of 2014, I ran my first half marathon. It was beautiful and exhilarating and one of the hardest things I'd ever done in my life. But it was also 13.1 miles of fun. And I slogged them in honor of my friend who died too soon.

Running didn't change my appearance much. I didn't lose 60 pounds. From the inside, though, I changed. Six months after running that half marathon, my body did something completely new and different. After twelve years of infertility, I was pregnant.

New life.

Becoming a runner was a life-altering experience for me. Each dull thud of my shoes against pavement carried me closer to the confidence and self-satisfaction that being a runner provided. The old me, the one

I'd given up on, was still in there.

I just had to run far enough to find her.

~Kelly A. Smith

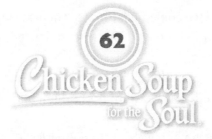

62

Bounce and Sway

There was a time in history, a long time ago,
when the bounce and sway of a woman's hips
was considered so beautiful that they set it
to music and made a dance out of it.
~Carolena Nericcio-Bohlman

The drummer in the corner of the room was lost in her own world. I sat on the floor and watched the women, who would eventually become my "tribe," enter one by one.

This was new to everyone and we all looked a little nervous, if not shy. Belly dancing would make us anything but shy or nervous. And over the course of this class, we would find a sisterhood in this dance we were about to share.

Our instructor, Kym, was petite and kind. She asked us to stand evenly spaced, feet hip-distance apart, with our bare feet rooted to the ground feeling the earth beneath us.

The drummer continued to play while we warmed up.

Class started with Kym moving her body in ways I didn't think were possible for me. It was hypnotic to watch. Then it was our turn. As a class, we tried our best to copy a few of the basic moves she had demonstrated. It was very strange to move this way, but once we got the hang of it, we blossomed as dancers.

The class ended as it would each week, with all of us gathering in a large circle around the room. Kym moved to the center and danced in front of us, and we copied her moves. Then she tagged each person to take the spot in the center. That woman danced, showing her own moves.

At first, this was difficult. But we all grew more confident over time, and it helped that we were not judgmental of each other, just loving and encouraging.

I am by no means a big girl; I am not perfect either. But this dance wasn't about being perfect or what society says is perfect. It was about celebrating our curves and diversity. I called us the Sacred Feminine Tribe, as we found acceptance for all our differences and came together to share in this ancient dance.

> *The most liberating thing for me was finding the courage to dress for class in the traditional clothing of a belly dancer.*

As the weeks turned into months, it was amazing to see the transformation in all of us. We became confident ladies celebrating the movements our bodies had learned. It wasn't anything risqué or sexual.

The most liberating thing for me was finding the courage to dress for class in the traditional clothing of a belly dancer. I became adept at sewing amazing outfits, from coin bras to flamenco style tops and flouncy skirts that billowed when I spun around, to the genie type pants normally worn — all of it was empowering.

The dance captivated, wowed, beguiled, and it gave me permission to be in command of the space I occupied as a female.

Because of belly dance, I understood that my body is unique and beautiful. And through this ancient and very proud form of celebration, I became more me than I ever thought possible.

~B. R. Dunkelman

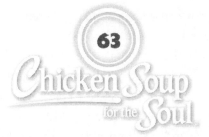

63

Swimming Toward Confidence

To all girls with butts, boobs, hips and a waist, put on a
bikini — put it on and stay strong.
~Jennifer Love Hewitt

ood for you," said the lean, middle-aged woman in the two-piece swimsuit as I walked by. "I see you out here swimming laps practically every day." I smiled politely and thanked her, then quickly made my way to the changing room.

It was mid-August and she was probably the fifth or sixth person that summer to make this type of comment to me. I was one of a handful of people who went to the lake almost every day to swim laps and I'd never heard anyone compliment the other swimmers on their dedication. If I had to guess, I would say that if I had weighed 120 pounds no one would have commented. But as someone who weighed more than twice that, I'm sure I stood out.

More than likely these people were well meaning, but whenever someone would say "Good for you" or "Way to go" I would hear: "Wow… you're pretty active for a 'fat' girl!"

A few summers before, these types of comments would have bothered me a lot more. Actually, a few summers before I wouldn't even have considered swimming at that lake.

Not that I wouldn't have loved to. Ever since I was old enough to walk, the water was my favorite place. When I was young and my parents would take me to the lake, I got annoyed when other kids wanted me to play in the sand or on the playground. We had this huge body of water to play in. Why would we want to be on the shore?

At that age, I wasn't embarrassed to be seen in a swimsuit. I was a chubby kid, but there were other chubby kids. It didn't seem to matter.

As a teen I was more self-conscious. I would still enjoy a swim, but I was quick to reach for a cover-up or a towel to wrap around myself as soon as I emerged from the water.

> *Even in regular clothes, I sometimes felt self-conscious — like everyone was looking at how big I was and silently judging me.*

By the time I reached adulthood, being seen in public in a swimsuit was out of the question. Even in regular clothes, I sometimes felt self-conscious — like everyone was looking at how big I was and silently judging me. They may not have been, but perception is reality. Wearing a swimsuit in public would leave me way too exposed.

It was a little easier when I was around people I trusted. My friend, Dirk, had a pool in his back yard and he could occasionally convince me to stop over and take a dip. One hot summer day, when I was thrilled at the thought of spending some time in the water, my heart sank as I pulled into Dirk's driveway. His sweet but stunningly gorgeous (and thin) sister, Casey, was there.

"Hurry up and get changed, Em," Dirk called out. "We're ready to get in the pool."

"You guys go ahead. I'm not really feeling it today," I said.

Dirk, always the straight shooter, rolled his eyes and looked at his sister.

"She doesn't want to be in front of you in her swimsuit," he told her.

"Are you serious?" Casey said as she walked over to me. "That is stupid. Get changed and let's go."

I reluctantly did as she said. I wasn't comfortable with it, but it was a blazing hot day and I hated to miss out. As we splashed around in the cool water that afternoon, it hit me — I was constantly missing out. For years I had been avoiding one of my favorite activities because

I was afraid of the way other people would look at me.

A few weeks later I worked up the nerve to go to the lake. I stood on the shore and took a deep breath before pulling off my clothes and darting into the water as quickly as I could. I felt a little strange and on display just bobbing around in the water so I headed to the area roped off for lap swimmers.

The muscles in my arms and shoulders ached that evening, but it was a good kind of pain. I went back a few days later and before I knew it, I was swimming almost daily.

Not only was I thrilled to be back in the water again, but I loved the way the exercise made me feel.

I may never be 120 pounds, but I'm mostly okay with that. To say I never feel self-conscious would be a lie, but learning all of the things my body can do, I find I'm a lot more comfortable in my own skin.

A couple of months after my brief conversation with the woman at the lake, I switched to swimming in the indoor pool at the local YMCA.

"Wow, you've been at it for almost an hour," said the man in the next lane. "You are really an inspiration."

"Thanks," I said with more confidence than I ever would have had years ago. "You seem to be working really hard, too. Great job."

~Emily Canning-Dean

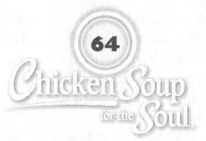

64

The Walk and Talk Diet

Friendship is born at that moment when one
person says to another, "What! You too? I
thought I was the only one."

~C.S. Lewis

I met my friend Tina while we were both prying our screaming sons off our legs for their first day of kindergarten. She looked a lot like me — hair pulled back into a ponytail, T-shirt and comfy pants, with a little extra padding.

We realized we were experiencing our first taste of freedom with our youngest sons in school. "Would you like to go for a walk?" was my creative pick-up line. She fell for it, and that began the walk that launched a thousand walks, and the start of our "Walk and Talk Diet."

We were two chubby young moms, desperate for exercise and the few hours of freedom that having kids in school allowed us.

Over the past ten years Tina and I have walked twice a week, the same long neighbourhood route, after getting our kids off to school. Our walk is about 4.5 kilometres and ends at the local McCafé with a coffee reward for our labours (and sometimes a muffin to go with it). We figure we walk about 500 kilometres a year, or 83,2000 steps (according to our Fitbits). This adds up to almost 5,000 kilometres over ten years. (Please don't check my math, it's not my strong point!)

We walk through the heat, snow, ice, mud, and PMS. The Walk and Talk Diet hasn't really given us sleek svelte shapes, but it has improved our lives in so many other ways.

In the beginning, we were both desperate to lose the baby fat we'd gained having kids — especially now that our youngest were five years old. Over the years, one or both of us has been on some sort of diet to lose weight. We've walked through the "Cleansing Diet," the "800 Calorie Diet," the "Starve and Be Miserable Diet," and the "Just Eat and Be Happy Diet."

We tried weighing ourselves each week and throwing five dollars into a pot. The one who lost the most weight would get the money. Tina lost a pound or two, and used the money for a weekend away where she raved about the food for weeks.

We often talk about recipes. It's smart to discuss food when you're out walking and not even close to your refrigerator. Tina loves to eat at restaurants and sometimes our entire walk entails long descriptions of her latest dinner. "You should have seen the garlic pasta with roasted chicken dripping with mozzarella cheese and fresh herbs... and the thickest yogurt raspberry smoothies! For dessert, chocolate blondie sundaes dripping with caramel and chocolate sauce!"

The Walk and Talk Diet is about fresh air and exercise, friendship, and a counseling session all rolled into one.

By the time I get home I am ravenous!

The truth is, we started out walking as chubby young moms determined to get fit, and we're still walking as chubby middle-aged moms, but we are much more content with ourselves.

The Walk and Talk Diet is about fresh air and exercise, friendship, and a counseling session all rolled into one. Between the two of us, we have seven kids, and we've walked and talked each other through many years of issues — someone is always getting into trouble, graduating, and getting married. Her wisdom has kept me from offering up my kids for adoption many times.

We've walked through renovations on both our houses, turning forty, motorcycle lessons and accidents, husbands' illnesses and job losses, and being the generation between our teenagers and aging parents.

One day Tina decided we needed to start running. We invested in matching yoga pants and jackets (much to my teenage daughter's embarrassment), and decided to run from one telephone pole to the next, walk to the next pole and then run again at the next. That run from the first telephone pole to the next was the most excruciating marathon in the universe! That was the extent of our running career and we resorted to walking again.

What began as a simple walk has now turned into a necessity, a vital part of our lives. As the kids head out the door, we meet and begin our trek through the neighbourhood. As an added benefit, we see things others miss: Houses that are doing interesting renovations, teenagers skipping school, dogs running loose. If you give us an address, we can give you a full rundown of the type of house, who we think lives there and any exterior improvements we would make.

We live in a small town and are often recognized with horn honks, waves or people saying "I see you out walking a lot…" I hope we're not becoming one of the town characters that everyone knows about, like "The man who walks through town singing opera," or "The lady with the giant red hat who rides her pink bike in the middle of the road."

We're probably known as "The Chubby Twin Walkers — who have walked for years, but still look the same size."

One Christmas Eve, it was our regular Monday to walk, and we were both at home swamped with last minute cookie baking and toy wrapping. I got a frantic call: "Lori, can we PLEASE walk today?" We piled on our warmest coats, trudged through the snow and collapsed in front of the fake fireplace at McCafé, happy to ignore our "to-do lists" at home.

In recent years we talk more about acceptance, gratitude, and of not worrying about the numbers on the scale. One day, as we walked, I looked over at Tina and confessed, "You know, I wouldn't like you any better if you were skinny. I like you just the way you are." After she slugged me in the arm, she admitted, "I like you chubby, too." Over the years of walking and probably about fifty different diets, we realized a great truth. Our size didn't matter to our friendship. We were growing to accept who we were as women, and as friends. We were making peace with the bodies we had been given. Maybe if our diets had worked in the beginning, we would have stopped walking together.

The Walk and Talk Diet is for everyone. All you need is a comfy pair of shoes and a friend who likes to walk and talk (or listen, depending on which one of you has the gift of gab). Tina has heard the worst parts of my life, and walked me — literally — through some very emotional times. I can't imagine my life without our walks.

I hope that in another ten years when all our kids have grown and left the nest, Tina and I will still be on our Walk and Talk Diet. I'm sure by then we will have walked ourselves through a lot more of life's ups and downs. Maybe we will even have lost a pound or two, but that doesn't really matter, now, does it?

~Lori Zenker

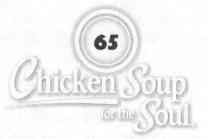
Strength to Be Strong

Take care of your body. It's the only place
you have to live.
~Jim Rohn

It's 7 A.M. and I am standing with 160 pounds on my back. I squat one. Two. Three. I slam the barbell back onto the rack and load on more weight. The sweat dripping down my face reminds me that I am a strong woman.

I move to the deadlift station. Can I handle eight sets of deficit deadlifts after ten sets of heavy squats? Of course I can. I am strong.

Rewind to before I discovered lifting. Growing up, I was constantly scrutinized. My family moved to America from Romania. Sometimes they would tell me that I had gotten fat or that I had a huge pimple on my face. They would pat my belly and ask, "When's the baby due?" or "Did the shirt come with the stomach?" They thought they were being funny, that they were showing affection for me.

I didn't care when I was growing up — at least, I thought I didn't care. I would get upset when the boy I had a crush on had a crush on other girls, but I never thought it was because I was ugly or fat.

But then, as adolescence went on, I started to believe that I *was* ugly and fat because I had acne and I couldn't fit in my neighbor's clothes. Other girls around me started "dating" boys, while I couldn't even get someone to come over and jump on my trampoline with me, let alone take me to a movie or give me a scandalous hug and kiss on the cheek.

Fast forward to college. At this point, I had alternated between being skinny and fit or being fat and lazy. I had gone through periods when I wouldn't eat anything and periods when I would eat everything. I felt like I couldn't control how I felt about myself because I couldn't control how I looked.

I started working out and logging my food. Counting calories isn't bad as long as you are eating enough to sustain you. I wasn't starving myself; I was just making sure I wasn't eating so much that I was gaining weight again.

I would go to the gym and lift or I would go on runs. But I never felt like a real runner or a bodybuilder or anything that actually made me feel good about myself. I was too focused on trying to fit into smaller pants and making sure I would never have to buy a shirt bigger than a size small.

Though I was technically eating right and exercising, and I had lost some weight, I still hated my body. If I weighed in one week and I had only lost half a pound instead of a full one, or if I didn't lose anything at all, I would binge on frosted sugar cookies, rationalizing that dieting wasn't working anyway. I fluctuated between eating right and eating poorly, and I was really hard on myself when my mile time was slower than the day before or when I failed a set of squats on a weight that I should have been able to do.

> *My focus is on being strong. Strength in the weight room can lead to strength in all areas of life.*

After a while, I stopped doing my weight loss program. I would go to the gym with my boyfriend, who is a powerlifter and personal trainer, and I would do his workout instead.

Being able to say I weigh a certain amount would probably feel pretty good. But saying I can squat 185 pounds is a completely different feeling. I weigh about the same as I did when I started, but now I have more muscle and my weight is distributed differently.

My focus is on being strong. Strength in the weight room can lead to strength in all areas of life. If I can lift hundreds of pounds, I can handle rejection. If I can lift hundreds of pounds, I can handle the uncertainty of the future, and I can definitely handle not having society's idea of the "perfect" beach body because that is not what matters. Now I know I can handle anything.

Focusing on my strength rather than my weight has actually helped me manage my weight. When I lift more, I can eat more and without gaining weight. By lifting, I build muscle and redistribute my weight. My legs are still big and my thighs still touch, but now my quad muscles show when I'm standing and I'm proud that they're so big.

It's 7 A.M. and I stand with 160 pounds on my back. Every squat is a reminder that I am beautiful, that I deserve to feel beautiful, and that above all else, I am a strong woman.

~Nicole Christine Caratas

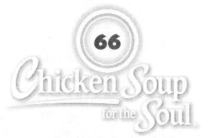

66

My Aha Moment

You yourself, as much as anybody in the entire
universe, deserve your love and affection.
~Buddha

I had confidence in myself growing up. I was confident that I was a good friend, good daughter and good sister. I was confident I could get good grades in school and meet expectations. I was confident in my ability to be a good athlete and take my athletic abilities to the next level. I was confident after college that I would navigate my way through the adult world and be responsible. And I was confident that I was a good woman who helped others.

But there was one thing I was not confident about — my body.

I was always tall and curvy but never accepted my shape, the beautiful body I was given, the way it was. The norm seemed to be what I saw on commercials and in the advertisements in all the stores.

Growing up, it was rare to see me in a dress. The few times I did wear one, my friends told me how wonderful I looked, that I was stunning. I didn't believe them. I thought: *I will never look like the girls that get dolled up with make-up and have great dresses, shoes and hair. That's not me.*

Instead, I wore what was comfortable, usually my basketball clothes and sports gear. I knew I wouldn't be noticed as much or critiqued about my body because it was hidden away under my Nike gear.

Fast forward to my adult life. One Saturday night, a few years ago, my friends asked me to go to a concert. It was my favorite artist but I said I couldn't make it. Little did they know I declined because I didn't feel comfortable getting into my little black dress.

Then I had an *aha* moment. I was depriving myself of fun activities because I didn't want to be seen in a certain dress? Really? In that moment, I decided not to waste any more time playing the same old tape in my head. I decided that I would go out and do things that made me happy right then and there, not at some future time "when I'm the weight that I want to be."

> *I was depriving myself of fun activities because I didn't want to be seen in a certain dress? Really?*

I called my friends and went out. I had the best time and I never looked back.

After that day, I started to wear clothes that hugged my curves and dresses that made me feel great. I was embracing my shape… finally! I still loved to lounge around in sports gear and sweats (who doesn't?) but I wasn't hiding under layers anymore.

Women even started asking where I got my clothes. They asked me what had changed and how I had found my new confidence. I started telling them my story, from the beginning to end.

"Wow," they'd say. "I wish I could feel that way about myself."

But why can't they? They can.

Today, I make my living as a plus-size model. I'm still no fashionista, but I know my confidence shines through.

I will never again let a negative thought take life's happy moments away from me.

~Devon Kab

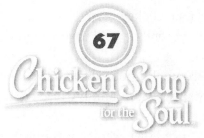

67

When Life Throws You Curves

Cultivate your curves — they may be dangerous,
but they won't be avoided.
~Mae West

I sat at the bar, nervously peeling the label off the bottle. I checked my phone for the fiftieth time in two minutes.

We agreed on 6:30 P.M. It was now 6:25. I was already worried that he would stand me up.

I hadn't been on a date in months, and I was the one who suggested it. He seemed like a nice guy on the dating site. He was funny, he texted or called when he said he would, and we had chemistry. But meeting face to face… this could make or break our fledgling relationship.

At least he knew I was a size 20. That was a real turn-off for a lot of guys on dating sites, but Chris seemed okay with it. He was on the larger side himself, which was more than fine with me — I preferred dating teddy bears.

Picking imaginary lint off my sweater, I reflected on the times I thought my size would be a barrier to doing the things I wanted.

My mind drifted to my undergraduate days, when a group of French exchange students begged me to go out with them.

"C'mon! Let's go salsa dancing!"

"Why would I want to do that?" I replied. The only salsa I ever came in contact with was on the nachos I ate. Not to mention, I could barely dance the Hokey Pokey.

"Just come. We promise you'll have a good time. There will be a lot of guys there."

My ears perked up. I supposed I could go if boys would be there. I donned my new strapless, formfitting black dress, unsure of what I would encounter.

What I experienced that evening was unlike anything I ever had before. Latin music pulsed all around us: Elvis Crespo, Marc Anthony, and Enrique Iglesias. I had little trouble picking up steps to merengue and salsa. I may have stepped on a few toes and kept my eyes glued to the floor to ensure I had the basic steps correct, but wrapped in the arms of handsome men, swaying my hips, and twirling as they led, I never felt more powerful in my curves than I did that night.

That was the beginning of many nights dancing.

After I graduated college, I secured a position in France teaching English, and it was one of the best years of my life. I fell in love with teaching and worked on building great relationships with my students and fellow English teachers.

But one day I was passing a classroom when I heard one of the teachers, a cynical man named Pierre-Yves, say in a heavy, Franco-British accent, "Be careful not to eat too much fast food. You don't want to end up fat like Americans. I mean, Miss Kontor is about the size of Godzilla!"

My face burned. I burst through the classroom door and in perfect French, said, "So is my name Miss Kontor or Godzilla? I'm confused."

His face turned crimson. In English he stammered, "Miss Kontor, of course."

I shook my head and continued in French: "If you're going to insult me, you can at least be honest about it."

"I meant it as a joke," was his feeble excuse.

"No one's laughing," one of the students piped up.

"Yeah, we like Miss Kontor," said another. And then more spoke up. "She's nice to us!"

"Who cares if she is bigger? She treats us better than you."

I looked Pierre-Yves square in the eyes. "I weigh more than you, but at least I conduct myself like a professional. I don't insult other teachers in front of students." I spun around on my heels and marched off, straight to the language department chair to file a complaint. I heard hooting and hollering behind me as the students continued their attack on Pierre-Yves.

After my adventures in Europe, I settled down to the life of an American schoolteacher. I spent over sixty hours a week planning lessons and grading papers. After a couple of years, my body was screaming for rest and rejuvenation. I signed up for yoga classes at a local gym.

I had never taken a yoga class in my life. I looked around at the thinner women and, in awe at the poses they contorted themselves into, I felt woefully inadequate.

> *As the weeks progressed, I realized I was just as flexible as the other women.*

But as the weeks progressed, I realized I was just as flexible as the other women, sometimes even more so. I could sit cross-legged with my knees touching the floor. I could arch my body up into a perfect half-circle. I could do headstands — something I could never do in the hundreds of gym classes I was forced to endure as a girl.

Yoga made me feel strong, centered, and serene — words I had never used to describe myself before. My body was capable of more than I had imagined.

I had always wanted to jog, but I never thought I could because I was too big. But my cousin told me about Couch to 5K, a program that teaches you how to run in nine weeks. You start by running in one-minute bursts, then walking. Eventually, you run longer periods of time until you can run an entire 5K race. Though I hated rising at 5:30 A.M., I loved jogging in the dark, starlit dawns. I lost a dress size in a matter of weeks. Within four months, I ran my first 5K and I've run three more since.

Though my time is never fast and I often place last in my age group, I know I lap everyone who's still sitting on the couch and I'm pushing my body to do something I always wanted to do. I continue to jog to this day.

I snapped out of my daydream and looked toward the door to see

Chris, holding a white carnation — the symbol for sweetness. He was way cuter than his picture, and I actually stopped breathing.

As soon as he saw me, his eyes lit up.

"Annie! It's so nice to finally meet you!" He slid into the seat next to mine and offered me the carnation. No man had ever given me flowers before.

Chris was the real deal. And my curves weren't about to hold me back!

~Annie Kontor

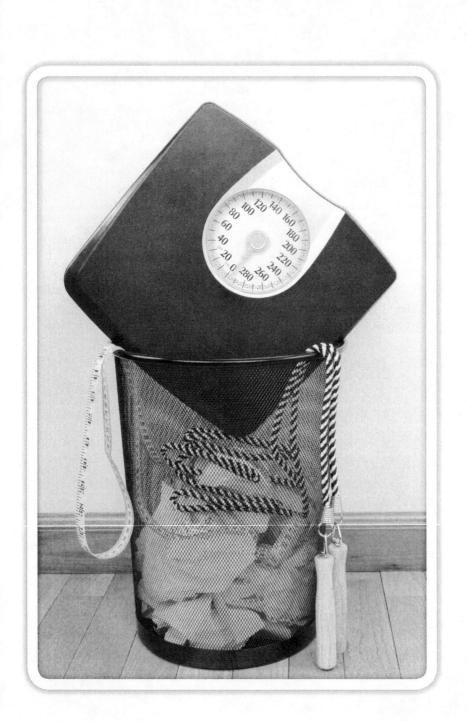

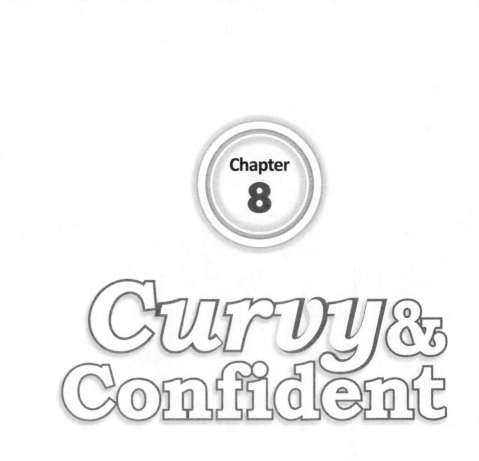

Chapter 8

Curvy & Confident

My Miraculous Body

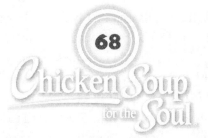

68

The Skin I'm In

To love oneself is the beginning of a life-long romance.
~Oscar Wilde

The women on my mother's side of the family have never been petite. I watched my mom struggle with her body and self-image for years. It confused me, because I thought she was beautiful. In college I was curvy, but thin — I never struggled with weight myself.

Then came marriage, and babies! I put on a whopping 60 pounds when I was pregnant with my son. Those curves got a little curvier! When my son was three I worked hard and lost weight before my thirtieth birthday, getting back down to my college size. Then came baby number two! I gained over 50 pounds with that pregnancy. I felt like a yo-yo. In my early thirties now, that weight was harder to lose.

After some health issues and discouragement over my figure I had an "aha!" moment. I realized I am not the sum total of all my parts; my dress size or my hips do not define who I am. My body is a gift. It's how I engage with the world and it deserves respect.

My body had made space for life. It had incubated miracles. It nurtured the tiny humans I loved. I started seeing myself in a different light. My arms held babies when they were sad, or sleepy, or in need of affection. My lap had grown wider, with plenty of room for two crowding in for story time.

Until motherhood woke me up to the amazing things my body could do I had taken it for granted. Then, I underwent a rebirth. Each stretch mark and "flaw" tells a story. My body allows me to experience beauty, show emotion, feel comfort, worship, create, move, thrive, live, love. I had missed that truth in my twenties.

> *I've learned to watch how I talk about my body because I know my daughter is watching.*

I've learned to watch how I talk about my body because I know my daughter is watching. She'll need to know how to make peace with her own figure one day. I want her to see her body as more than an ornament, more than a fashion statement. I want her to know that her body is a miracle. That it's made to express and receive love.

I am curvy, weighing the most I ever have. I love healthy food and taking a good long walk. My fortieth birthday is around the corner. I may lose weight before it's here. I may not. But either way I know I will embrace it with confidence.

~Beck Gambill

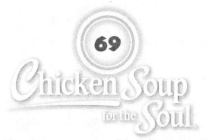

69

To Have and To Hold

Who looks outside, dreams; who looks inside, awakes.
~Carl Gustav Jung

A s soon as I announced my engagement, my mom wanted to go dress shopping. She didn't have a dream wedding with her own true love, my amazing stepdad, and she'd been dreaming about seeing me glide down the aisle in a sea of tulle, lace, satin, and sparkle for a long time. The problem was, I was less than enthusiastic about the prospect of trying on wedding dresses.

Each time Mom suggested a trip to the bridal boutique, I'd make an excuse: I was busy, I had to work, or I had to write a paper for school. Unfortunately, none of these was true. I dreaded looking for a wedding dress because I was "too fat."

I was one of the last of my friends to get married, something I attributed to my weight, of course. I didn't conform to society's idea of what a bride should look like (even though my fiancé thought I looked fine), so I figured that the search for the perfect wedding dress would be torture.

I imagined derisive stares from salesladies, painful girdles and corsets squeezing me like a stuffed sausage. I shuddered thinking about what size wedding dress they'd have to drag out of some dusty closet to accommodate me. Everyone in the store would snicker behind my back and pity me, the chubby bride. It was as if I didn't deserve to get married because I wasn't tiny.

So I went on a diet. That was, after all, what every girl was supposed to do the second she got engaged, right? I know all my friends did, even the slender ones. Dieting was pretty much a mandatory part of wedding planning: get engaged, choose a venue, agonize over bouquets and color schemes, and starve yourself to death. I would have been remiss if I didn't at least suffer through a few juice cleanses, so I started low-carbing, walking, and going to the gym.

But then I got sick. I'm not talking about a little cold here; this was serious. I had a large tumor on my thyroid, something called a toxic adenoma, and it was making me feel terrible.

> My tumor was a wake-up call, showing me how my self-consciousness was preventing me from enjoying what should have been the happiest time of my life.

On top of that, the tumor needed to be treated with radiation at a cancer center, so the months before my wedding filled up with doctor appointments, scary tests, results I didn't want to hear, and more needles than I could possibly count.

Suddenly, table settings, guest lists and the font on my invitation didn't seem important. And you know what? Neither did my weight.

When I went to the cancer center, I saw patients far sicker than me — people who were frail from illness, people who might die. I felt thankful and lucky — my belly rolls, dimpled thighs, and wide, flat butt didn't seem so bad when I viewed my flab as an indication that I was alive, that I was ultimately going to be okay, and that I was not wasting away from disease.

I didn't lose weight before my wedding. In fact, I gained a few pounds. Some of the medications slowed my metabolism and made me bloated, but by then, I didn't care. Getting sick taught me not to take my body and my life for granted and not to hate myself. My tumor was a wake-up call, showing me how my self-consciousness was preventing me from enjoying what should have been the happiest time of my life. I vowed from then on to celebrate — and, to have a macaroni and cheese bar at the reception!

Dress shopping, that once feared chore, turned into something of a miracle. The afternoon I found my wedding dress, I was surrounded by people who loved and cared for me in sickness and in health, regardless of my size.

When I zipped up my gown for the first time, the size on the tag was the furthest thing from my mind. I felt beautiful and joyful. My entire perspective on life had changed and it was freeing. All I wanted to do was dance.

My husband and I had the greatest wedding. Sure, my cheeks were round and my upper arms look as plump as canned hams in every photo. One of my great-aunts mentioned my size and asked if I was pregnant, but I laughed her off. I'd learned that a wedding isn't about what you look like; it's about gathering your favorite people together to celebrate love and have a good time.

I savored every second of the meaningful ceremony and the raucous party that followed. And yes, I ate plenty of that mac and cheese and the delicious cake we'd picked out without a shred of regret. I didn't care that I wasn't 30 pounds thinner. No one has ever once gone to a wedding and left saying: "Well, it was a nice party with a fantastic DJ and an impressive buffet, but I would've had a better time if the bride had been skinnier."

My body wasn't meant to suffer in order to conform to some arbitrary standard of what a bride ought to look like. My body carries my spirit so that I can live this beautiful life to the fullest, enjoying and celebrating every second — grateful that my arms, however chunky, can embrace the man I love.

~Victoria Fedden

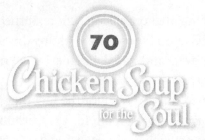

70

A Fish Out of Water

If you judge a fish by its ability to climb a tree, it will
live its whole life believing that it is stupid.
~Albert Einstein

I was a tomboy. I liked being outside getting dirty and playing baseball in the street. I had a wicked throwing arm — no matter how far the ball went down the street, I could throw it back to home plate.

I loved climbing trees, building forts, catching fish in the creek and rescuing wounded animals. But my favorite activity was scavenging scrap wood to make a raft to float down the creek behind our house. When it reached the river, I'd jump off and swim to shore. I loved the water.

When my father was stationed in Hawaii with the Army, our family would go to the beach on weekends. We kids mostly played on the beach or waded in the water. I was six when my father told me there were hundreds of colorful tropical fish past the breakers, on a reef half a mile from shore. I wanted to see them.

"You aren't strong enough," my father said. "If you are able to swim out there, I'll go with you."

He promptly forgot that he made this promise, but I didn't.

When school was out, my mother took us four kids to the base pool nearly every day. There were three pools: One for babies, one for kids playing, and the adult lap pool. I wanted to swim in the adult pool. I wanted to practice so I could swim a half-mile to see the fish.

At seven, I asked the lifeguard every day to let me swim in the adult pool. Hardly any adults swam there during the day because they were at work. I guess the lifeguard finally got tired of me asking because one day he said if I could swim 200 yards without stopping, he'd give me an adult pass and I'd be able to swim there any time I wanted!

I practiced in the play pool for two weeks. When I took the swim test, I kept swimming until the lifeguard finally grabbed me and stopped me. I got my swim pass! From that day on, I swam every chance I had. I grew stronger and started to have visible muscles. When it was time to swim out to the reef, my father was the one who couldn't make it. His friend swam with me the rest of the way.

I matured early, and by ten I had the height and figure of a grown woman. I was sensitive about my mature body and hated the way boys looked at me. I started swimming with a T-shirt on. Other fifth grade girls didn't experience this problem so they made fun of me. They couldn't imagine how self-conscious I was about my body. By seventh grade, I was so shy that I rarely looked anyone in the eye.

My love for swimming continued, but I noticed that the other girls on the swim team stayed thinner and significantly less curvy than me. I didn't let that keep me from competing, but between races I'd huddle under two towels. It was lonely being so different.

I tried different sports — track, softball, kickboxing, cycling and racketball — and I was usually the curviest girl there, too. My athletic ability was often overlooked because of my body shape. As an adult, a co-worker asked me to be on the company's co-ed softball team and I was thrilled.

"You don't have to play; just sit on the bench," he said. Apparently, they needed another woman or they had to forfeit the game.

I sat on the bench and watched as the team dropped fly balls and overthrew the bases. When our team was down by four runs in the seventh inning, they put me in. I made two outs at first base, and clobbered the ball for a triple with the bases loaded, adding three points to our score. My co-workers were in shock. I could play; I just didn't *look* like I could play.

After college, I taught swimming. I loved working with kids, but it hurt every time parents asked for a different teacher before I even worked with their child. They assumed I was a bad swim teacher because of my full figure. The other teachers "looked like swimmers." By the end of the four-week beginner class, my students could swim in the adult pool while the other kids were still doing the dog paddle. After that first summer, I always had a waiting list of students for my classes.

I was also the head coach for several year-round competitive swim teams and once again, parents walked out before their child even swam with me. It happened so often that by the time I was thirty I had a full-blown case of body shame. Getting into the water to work with the kids on stroke technique became difficult for me.

> *I realized how beautiful and strong my body must be to this young girl who wanted to be a swimmer like me.*

I had a natural feel for the water. I was a born swimmer. I could teach anyone of any age to swim well. It was both a source of great joy and pain for me that my strong, athletic body was considered "fat" by so many people.

One day, after swim practice, one of the nine-year old girls on my team said she wanted to have a body just like mine when she grew up. Tears welled in my eyes.

"I want my thighs to have big muscles like yours some day."

I realized how beautiful and strong my body must be to this young girl who wanted to be a swimmer like me. She saw my life, energy and joy when I swam. She saw my passion for the sport when I coached her. I was a role model of what a swimmer was supposed to be. She, and the other swimmers on my team, didn't see me as a "fat" woman; they saw me as the athlete I was. I was still that seven-year old who swam a mile out and back to the reef to see the fish.

My body may be a liability on land but it is perfectly equipped for water. I was only fat when I wasn't in my natural element. I was only fat in the eyes of those I wasn't built for.

But I was built for this nine-year-old girl's eyes. I was built to show this future swimmer, who wanted to be just like me, that she could do anything. I was built to mentor and teach her to love herself. I was built to teach her how to get anything she worked hard for no matter what she looked like.

I was built to show her how to be the amazing woman she was built to be.

Just like me.

~Kathryn Lehan

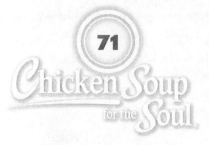

71

Shifted

The years teach much which the days never knew.
~Ralph Waldo Emerson

The sales clerk looked at me in the long gown I was trying on. "It's lovely on you," she said, but she didn't sound thoroughly convinced. "All you need is a little Spanx under it." Spanx, for those who don't know, is the skinless, boneless equivalent of your grandmother's boned and trussed girdle. I nodded dumbly. I didn't tell her I was already wearing Spanx!

I looked at my bulges, I mean curves, and did a quick calculation. I had two weeks before my special occasion. Even if I moved into the gym for two solid weeks it would not dislodge what had taken up squatter's rights on my body for twenty years. When the sales clerk turned her back I slipped out and grabbed the same dress in the next size up. It draped over my childbearing hips and I didn't have to hold my breath to get it zipped.

To be honest, I don't think I cared what size it was. What I was trying to avoid was looking "matronly." Heaven forbid, that I, a mother of four and a grandmother of five, should look matronly!

I well remember the first time I felt matronly. I was browsing the petunias for sale outside a neighborhood corner store. Thirty years old, with three little ones clinging to me and a fourth protruding from my maternity top, I wobbled around the annuals on display. Then I saw her, a nursing colleague of mine, my age, but slim-hipped and tiny-waisted, coming out of the store. She hopped on a red motorbike and sped off down the road. Norma looked like a young girl, slender and carefree. Suddenly I felt frumpy, lumpy and encumbered. She never even spoke to me. I was sure I looked so old and matronly she had not recognized me.

Life teaches us things in a funny way, so it was years before I gained a different perspective on that day. My children were all raised and I had gone back to nursing. There was my old colleague Norma, kindly orientating me to my new job. We were chatting and I mentioned how I had envied her that day when she didn't even see me and she looked so young and carefree.

I didn't tell her I was already wearing Spanx!

Norma explained. "I couldn't speak to you," she said, her eyes watering. "All I desperately wanted was a baby. And there you were, pregnant again, with all those little ones at your side. I took off fast before you could see my tears."

That was a shift in perspective.

I've learned to look for those ways to shift. My husband loves all things techy and recently bought a new digital scale that is smarter than the old clunker I had, and twice as mean. This new shiny, silvery thing is programmable, an awful word, which means that it tells you not only your weight, but also your percentage of body fat. My husband kindly put in my height and his and set the thing to remember it all. I was encouraged the next day to find out I weighed the same as a television super-model. But did shiny-scale compliment me? No. It flashed body-fat warning lights so urgently I expected to hear a siren go off as well. It wouldn't let me quite forget that I was only 5'4". So, I adjusted my "personal data" a teeny, tiny bit. Mr. Meany Scale now has me at 6'4" and an almost normal body fat percentage.

Now I laugh every time I get on that scale. Of course I know I am not 6'4" and nothing I do will make me taller. The weight? I have learned to be more realistic in my expectations. I walk. I bike. I eat a lot of green soups and tofu, but despite that I have seen that after a certain age things shift. And maybe that is appropriate. I think of things that used to cause me stress and now I just take them in stride.

I think of attitudes I've adjusted after hearing different sides of a story. I think of how the places I've been, the books I've read and the people I've met have changed me. Softened me. Broadened me. Perhaps, after all, my body is just trying to tell me it's okay to loosen up a bit. It's okay not to force fit myself into something not quite right for me. Everything shifts over time.

I learned to be grateful for my hands after seeing my sister's hand immobilized by a stroke. I learned to be satisfied with my God-given endowments when they nursed four babies and when several women very close to me, including my daughter, suffered devastating mastectomies. I learned to love my legs when I saw a friend with multiple sclerosis rely every day on her walker. I learned to appreciate my body when I began to realize, that despite its squeaks and creaks, its sags or bags, it has been my personal, living, breathing miracle and has faithfully served me all these years.

By the way, I wore that dress in the bigger size with such dazzlingly sexy shoes that no one could accuse me of looking the least bit matronly!

~Phyllis McKinley

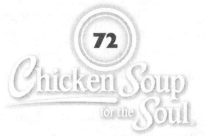

72

Skinny Doesn't Matter

Becoming acquainted with yourself is a price well
worth paying for the love that will really
address your needs.
~Daphne Rose Kingma

"**M**om, are you chubby or skinny?" My seven-year-old daughter studied me as if she'd been considering this question for some time.

I glanced at myself in the nearby mirror. I was somewhat chubby, still carrying an extra 15 pounds from my three pregnancies. In the past three years, I had also gained and lost 30 pounds from depression and a malfunctioning thyroid. And then came two miscarriages.

But now, three months after having my son, I was feeling pretty good — liking myself and getting back to who I wanted to be — in body and mind.

No, I wasn't the athletic, thin girl I was in my twenties. But here I was, three months postpartum, and down 20 pounds from where I was two years earlier. And besides, my health journey wasn't about the number on the scale. Even though I was heavier than I'd been pre-baby, I felt healthier than I had in decades, possibly ever.

I sat down on the bed beside my daughter and looked into her dark brown eyes. At seven, she was tall and thin. But she had a whole life ahead of her.

This was an important conversation. How I chose to see myself now would be reflected in how she and her sister saw themselves in the future. As a teacher I'd seen too many young girls obsess over their size no matter how small and thin they were.

"I like to think I'm neither, because honestly it doesn't matter," I said.

"Why do you work out so often then," she asked, "and get all excited about losing weight or about your clothes fitting?"

Kids were observant, and she was right. How did I explain to a seven-year-old that even though I was excited about fitting into my smaller clothes, being skinny wasn't important? Getting skinny wasn't why I was working out and eating better. I was doing it to be in a better place mentally.

> *How I chose to see myself now would be reflected in how she and her sister saw themselves in the future.*

"Your mind and your body are connected," I told her. "Before I had you kids, I used to go to the gym every week. Then after you kids were born, remember how we used to walk… and then when we moved here, we walked less? Around that time, I also got sad and kind of grouchy."

"How does that fit with being skinny?" she asked.

"It doesn't and that's the point. After I had your brother, I wanted to make working out a habit again, because it makes me feel better and happier. Working out is good for you because it's healthy for your body to not be overweight, but it also has huge mental benefits for your brain. And it gives you energy, which I need to keep up with the kids at work and the three of you. Working out makes my body stronger physically and mentally so I can be healthier — to be here for a long, long, long time with you, your sister, and brother."

"So you're skinny?" she asked. ("No!" I wanted to scream. Why was this so hard to explain to her? And how could I convince her to delete that word from her vocabulary?)

"Honey, being skinny or chubby — "curvy" is a better way to say it — doesn't matter. It's about feeling good in your own skin and loving your body and treating it well. Anytime you do something good for yourself or others, you feel good about it, right?"

"Yes," she replied. "Then, I should feel fantastic when I'm your age," she added, as she grinned and flexed her arm muscles, "since I started working out with you when I was seven!"

I chuckled as she ran out of the room, and then I looked in the mirror again.

I had lost myself for a while, but now I'd found my way back. Just in time for my girls to see me as the confident mom I am now rather than the lost one of before.

~Angela Williams Glenn

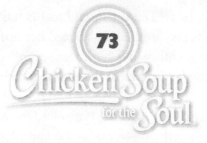
Exposed

*I'm one of the world's most self-conscious people. I
really have to struggle.*
~Marilyn Monroe

I took my shirt off in yoga class the other day. Get your mind
out of the gutter, there was no public indecency involved. It's
just that I usually hide my body under a double layer and
wear a tank top over my sports bra during yoga class.

Several of the women in the class were wearing midriff-baring
sports bras without covering up with a tank top, because it was hot. I
knew I'd feel better, too, without an unnecessary layer. Why did I feel
I had to hide myself? Why shouldn't I prioritize my physical comfort
over other concerns?

This might not seem like such a big deal to most people, but as
someone who has struggled with body image issues from early childhood, this was revolutionary. I realized that I did not have to hide. I
did not have to cover myself.

The teacher led us into a standing forward fold, bending at the
waist and reaching for our toes. I reached up and slipped my tank
top off over my head, exposing my belly and the biopsy scar left over
from a skin cancer scare. I did it while we were in a forward fold, so
that maybe none of the other students would notice.

My first thought was that I should have waited to remove my
shirt, as a forward fold is not the most flattering pose. I imagined my
rolls were on full display and my creamy white skin was glowing in

the dark. I immediately regretted my decision, but it would have been weird to put my tank top back on at that point.

A few moments later, as we settled into downward facing dog, I looked between my legs and noticed that the woman behind me, who had previously been wearing a tank top over her sports bra, had removed her tank top as well. She had been wearing it when we started, just like I had. My demonstration of self-love was contagious!

As the class progressed, I began to feel more comfortable with myself and my exposed midsection. My belly wasn't as big as I had imagined. That scar wasn't as noticeable as I thought. I bet most people wouldn't notice unless I pointed it out.

> *So why did I think they would be looking at me, judging me?*

I had chosen a spot away from the mirror, as usual, so I could concentrate on how I felt, and not what I looked like, doing the yoga poses. I thought about it and realized that I was not looking at anyone else. I didn't care what they looked like in their yoga clothes, exposed midriff or not. So why did I think they would be looking at me, judging me? I relaxed a little, and stopped obsessively sucking in my stomach.

By the end of class, I had progressed from wishing I could put my tank top back on, to kind of accepting my exposed belly, to actively loving myself. I shifted to plank pose and pulled my navel into my spine, pulling in my belly not because I was self-conscious, but to support the pose and work my abdominals. I thought about how strong I was and thanked my body for its amazing abilities. I occupied my space unapologetically. I allowed myself to take up as much room on my mat as possible as I lay down during *savasana* and took deep, belly-expanding breaths.

~Kathrine Conroy

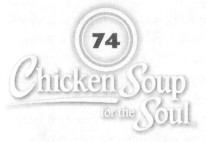

Look at Me

*There is a bit of insanity in dancing that does
everybody a great deal of good.*
~Edwin Denby

I'm at a healthy weight, normal for my height. I know that having a belly is natural. I know that I shouldn't compare myself to models in magazines. But still, when I look at myself, all I see is fat. I can't see the figure my college roommate is jealous of, but I eye her flat stomach with envy. I want to be pretty and feel pretty. I want to look at myself in the mirror and not hate the way I look. But I can't. I wear loose clothes and try to fade into the background.

But I'm tired of living this way and being this way. I want to change, yet I'm not sure how. A friend suggests belly dancing to me. She loves it and wants me to join. Belly dancing? I'd have to dance in front of people with my stomach exposed. I feel the anxiety immediately. But also, I feel a determination. I sign up.

I'm nervous at the first class, but at least we don't expose our bellies. We learn a few moves. I'm surprised by how fun it is, how much I'm enjoying moving my body like this. It feels so natural, so right. Except... shimmies make me feel ashamed of my body. As my hips shimmy up and down, so does all of my fat. No escape from the truth. But, I feel happy; everyone is so positive, so accepting.

Before our first performance, we are asked to say something that we love about ourselves. I say "my eyes" and almost believe it.

For our first performance, I assume few people will show up. My campus is conservative, so I'm thinking they'd be offended by the bellies we reveal. This soothes me, until it's our turn. My heart speeds up and adrenaline floods me, slamming into me, turning me into a shaking wreck. I want to cover myself, cover my belly, cover my fat.

Don't look at me.

It's time. We walk on stage, and I plaster a smile on my face. I look at the audience — it's jam-packed with strangers watching us, waiting. I want to hide my body.

Don't look at me.

The music starts and we dance. We turn and shimmy; I'm a well-oiled dance machine. My face hurts from smiling; just get me out of here. I feel like I'm going to cry.

Don't look at me.

The song finishes, and I want to run off the stage, but we walk. I cover up as soon as we're off. I'm shaking, not all of it from the fear. I realize that it was exciting. I want to do it again.

I look in the mirror and see my eyes. They're pretty.

The next performance, I decide to do a solo, to push myself. I want to feel that excitement again. I practice — my arms moving, their fat jiggling. I start to move them less; it's bad enough with my stomach, I don't want my arms to be stared at too.

My panic rises as I step onto the stage. I feel my smile wobble as I get into position. I try not to stare at all the faces upturned to me. I take a breath and feel my fat jiggle. I want to cringe off the stage, say it was all a mistake. There's no one else to distract the audience from me, from my fat. The music starts and I fall into familiar steps, acutely conscious of when my fat moves. Each jiggle makes me feel like I'm a dancing Jell-O. As I walk off stage, I hear their clapping. Maybe I wasn't a dancing Jell-O after all. Maybe, I was actually good.

I look in the mirror and see my arms. They are strong.

The next time we perform, I'm better prepared. I've practiced different moves, more complex. I feel my confidence growing, but still look down at my stomach and sigh. I do a solo again, this time with a shawl. Practice, practice, practice.

My Miraculous Body |

I stare out into the audience and feel the familiar fear fluttering in my stomach. It makes me tremble, makes my steps falter. I feel myself shrinking.

> *I dance, feeling sexy and desirable.*

But everything evaporates as soon as the music starts. I dance, feeling sexy and desirable. I don't see or feel my fat. All I feel is the music flowing through me and the strength and sensuality of my moves.

I don't want this to end. When the music cuts off I linger a moment on stage. Caught up in emotions I'd never thought I'd feel. I walk off stage. I don't cover up.

I look in the mirror and see a young woman. She has curves and she is beautiful.

~Maura Edwards

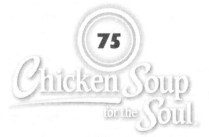

75

Take Center Stage

We have to learn to be our own best friends
because we fall too easily into the trap of
being our own worst enemies.
~Roderick Thorp

I am a charter member of the "Clean Your Plate, Children in Europe are Starving Club." As a first generation American, I heard that phrase constantly from my mother who emigrated from Bulgaria. I was led to believe that if I ate all my food, my distant cousins might somehow miraculously benefit. I needed little encouragement with the delicious cuisine served in my mother's kitchen.

Looking back to those days in the fifties, our daily fare was what restaurants now claim to be gourmet selections: succulent Bulgarian entrees such as roasted lamb, stuffed cabbage, and stuffed peppers; phyllo pastry filled with cheese; and baklava dripping with honey and walnuts. My taste buds were awakened and refined at an early age.

In grade school my brown-paper-sack lunch was easy to find when they opened the lunch cupboard doors. It was the one with a large grease stain on it from the leftovers from the previous night's dinner. No American peanut butter and jelly sandwich for me. My lunch was more like a juicy kielbasa.

In addition to developing a sophisticated palate, I also inherited Bulgarian genes, which meant I was short and a little stocky. As a teen, I often carried 10 to 12 pounds more than I should have. Spread over a mere five feet, there was not a lot of longitude to disperse the extra poundage. My thighs and hips attracted the extra calories and were a constant source of frustration to me as I saw my pear shape reflection in the mirror.

I probably first became conscious of my weight and the direct correlation it had to my self-esteem at age fourteen, my freshman year of high school. I don't think anyone would have suspected that there was a lot of negative self-talk going on in my head, as I participated fully in every activity, had many friends and even made the cheerleading squad. Only I knew how much more enjoyable those activities were when my weight was lower.

I soon discovered I had a summer weight and a winter weight. As spring arrived, I could shed 5 to 10 pounds easily by browsing through the Sears catalog and visualizing myself wearing those cute pedal pushers. Living near Lake Michigan and going to the beach often, the thought of my thunder thighs in a bathing suit helped me say "no" to French fries or an extra helping of a delicious moussaka.

However, as the autumn days grew short and dark, I inevitably gained back the 10 pounds. I'd be hiding them behind bulky sweaters all winter. My yo-yo dieting cycle was firmly established.

Through the years I tried every weight loss program: Weight Watchers, Nutri-System, Jenny Craig, Diet Center, Atkins, and Scarsdale. I was successful with each one, until I gained it all back.

Then, a few years ago, I had a revelation.

We were attending a Celebration of Life for a deceased family member and many of our old home movies were running. I saw my son's first birthday party and smiled again at the sight of a tow-headed little boy putting his entire hand in the icing. Then I saw myself on the screen, and I was shocked. I saw a somewhat attractive young mother, not the fat woman I thought I was.

In that moment, I grieved for all the occasions when I wasted negative energy because of 10 pounds. A mere 10 pounds often kept me from fully enjoying an experience because I thought I should have been thinner.

Today, at age seventy-five, I am still weight conscious, but more for health reasons than appearance. I am now the one preparing the delicious Bulgarian cuisine for my friends and family. I am twenty-five pounds more than my high school weight but active with tennis, pickle ball and golf. I often think of that home movie and vow to not let any negative self-judgment creep in as I participate fully in these activities.

The lesson I learned from that movie was that no one is judging me more harshly than I am. In fact, they are probably not even noticing my weight. Wasn't it Dr. Phil who said, "You wouldn't worry so much about what people think of you if you knew how little they do think of you. Most people are thinking of themselves."

I grieved for all the occasions when I wasted negative energy because of 10 pounds.

I'm starting a new club. Not a "clean your plate" club, but a "clean your mind of negative self-image" club. I want to embrace myself as I am, so my daughters and granddaughters will follow my example, learning to love their bodies and not be led astray by the unrealistic expectations of society.

When my family looks back at the movies we are making today, I want them to see a woman enjoying life to the fullest, not one hiding in the background for fear the camera might capture her flabby arms.

What do you want your loved ones to see in the movies and memories they will watch in years to come? I hope it is you center stage, participating in life with a beautiful smile, laughter and joie de vivre.

~Violetta Armour

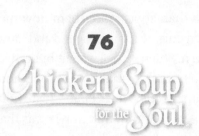

76

Becoming a Curvy, Confident Mom

Everybody has a part of her body that she doesn't like,
but I've stopped complaining about mine because I
don't want to critique nature's handiwork.
~Alfre Woodard

When I look at a portrait of my family today, I smile at the happy tableau — my husband and I stand proudly in the center of the photo with our beautiful daughters surrounding us. It's not what you would have seen a few years earlier.

Then, you would have seen our three beautifully outfitted little girls with matching bows in their hair standing around their father, who stood in the center in his neatly pressed shirt. Then, hiding in the background, you'd see me, wearing a sweatshirt and maybe mismatched socks. The expression on my face would have said it all: "I do not want to be in this picture."

Growing up, I was the only curvy member in my family. "It's just baby fat," my mother would say. "You'll grow out of it."

As a teenager I loved shopping at the local mall with my friends and longed to wear the same outfits as they did, but when I looked in the fitting room mirror those clothes never looked the same on my curvy frame.

"Someday, I hope I have a daughter. I will take her to the mall and make sure she has all the fashionable clothes I never got to wear," I used to tell myself.

"Someday shopping" would be fun in the future, and when it wasn't for me.

As fate would have it, I did not have one daughter... I had three! Dressing my girls became my full-time passion. I loved putting them in beautiful dresses; I wanted them to grow up with the confidence I never had and be proud of their appearance. I still didn't have that confidence. If I bought something for myself, it was at the last minute and whatever fit or hid the body I never came to terms with. *No one is looking at me anyway,* I thought.

As my girls grew they wanted to pick out their own clothes, which I knew was the natural order of things. However, I was surprised when they only wanted to wear their ripped jeans and T-shirts. On holidays our home became a battleground when my former little princesses wanted to put their hair in ponytails and just wear what was comfortable.

One time, I had a fight with my oldest daughter about why she couldn't wear her pants with a giant stain to our holiday dinner.

Frustrated, I confided to a friend about how I was feeling. I will never forget the way she gently put her hand over mine when she replied: "Raising a daughter," she said, "is a lot like looking in the mirror. We cannot give them what we are unwilling to give ourselves."

Her words hit home in a way I could not have expected. It was *me*, she pointed out, who was showing my girls what it was like to be a woman, and it was *my* behavior they would imitate. Not taking care of myself and how I looked was not taking care of them. If I did not love my curvy body, how could they grow to love the body types they were given?

My friend may have thought I'd be insulted by her words, but I was grateful. In fact, it was the highest compliment I had ever received, telling me that I was such a crucial element in their young lives.

After that day, I embraced the responsibility of being a mother to three teenage girls in a new way. I made peace with the woman in the fitting room mirror.

At the store, I did not buy the first thing that fit me anymore — I experimented with clothes that celebrated my curves instead of hiding them, and I tried colors other than black. I discovered I looked nice in patterns and bright hues. I enjoyed looking for accessories and punctuated my outfits with scarves and glittery earrings.

> *I experimented with clothes that celebrated my curves instead of hiding them, and I tried colors other than black.*

As the people around me noticed my efforts, they complimented me and it felt wonderful. Someone told me I looked taller, and that made me laugh. I knew I was walking with greater confidence and with my head held higher. Even my daughter's friends were excited by the changes they saw. I could tell my own girls were proud of how I looked.

My new behavior had a trickledown effect on my girls. As they moved through their teen years, my daughters began taking pride in their figures and spent more time caring for themselves and how they looked.

Today, if you look at our family pictures, you will see a curvy, confident mom standing in the center, smiling and happy to be there, with her proud family around her.

~Elizabeth Rose Reardon Farella

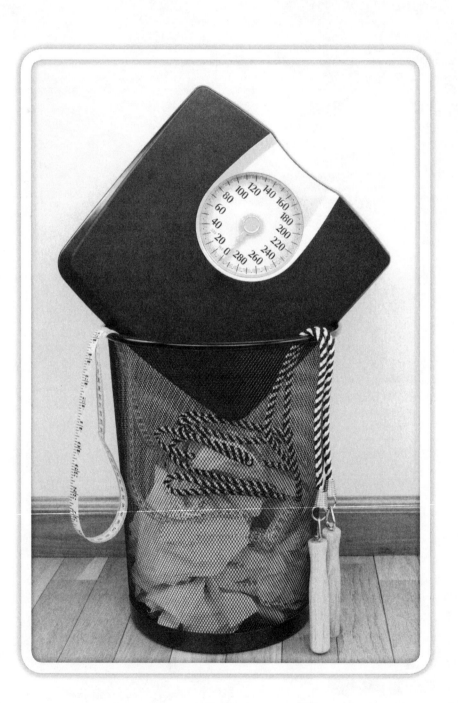

Curvy & Confident

Larger Size, Larger Life

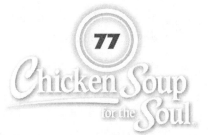

77

Thunder Thighs and All

I might have a little bit of cellulite. I might not be toned
everywhere. I might struggle in this area or that. But
accepting that just empowers me.
~Kim Kardashian, Harper's Bazaar

"**Y**ou want me to present myself half-naked to a bunch of strangers?" I asked my husband, Wayne, when he suggested I join his master's swim team.

"All body types are there," he said, knowing how self-conscious I was about my size. "And all ages and skill levels," he added, anticipating my next argument. "It's not about what you look like or how fast you swim. It's about getting in the water and enjoying some exercise."

Enjoy? When was the last time I enjoyed being in a bathing suit? Probably the last time I was thin, which was around age ten.

And when was the last time I swam laps? Had I ever? No.

My husband was the fish in our family. Growing up he'd spent summers at his neighborhood pool, competing on the community swim team, and in high school he was a lifeguard. As a kid, I was more the show-up, splash-around-when-I-got-hot, and then go-eat-snacks-on-my-towel type.

I'm not sure how he finally convinced me to go. I think it was the promise of the social aspect. I had just moved from Phoenix to Jacksonville to join him — he'd moved earlier for work — and I hadn't started working or making any friends yet.

"The team is great," he said. "They get together and have parties from time to time. They go out to eat after practices. Trust me. You'll like it."

It was something for us to do together as a couple. Sort of. He'd swim in a faster lane than I would, but we could talk driving to and from the pool. It might be fun.

If it weren't for the fact that I had to put on a bathing suit.

Which in and of itself, wasn't that bad. On the occasions we did something that called for a bathing suit, I kept my thighs covered with a sarong or shorts. That's what I was most embarrassed about — my thick, jiggly, cottage-cheese-stuffed, stretch mark-scarred thighs. All of me was chunky, but my thighs were the worst. They were hideous and I knew it. I was doing the world a public service concealing them.

Now my husband was asking me to expose them for public viewing. It made my stomach churn.

"Give it a try one time," he said. "That's all I'm asking. If you're miserable, I'll never ask you to go again."

I gave in, because my heart knew how lucky I was to have a husband who wanted to spend time with me. Thunder thighs and all.

My stomach was in knots all the way to that first practice. To my relief, a lot of people were already in the pool swimming warm-up laps when we arrived. Wayne introduced me to the coach, Walter.

"I've never done this before," I confessed. "I'm afraid I'll be slow."

"No problem," said Walter. "We've got a lane for all speeds. Let's try this one for starters. See how it fits."

He led me to the first lane. A lady in her seventies was at the wall adjusting her goggles. "Joan, this is Courtney. She's a newbie. Show her the ropes, will you?"

"Be glad to," said Joan. "Grab a kickboard and hop on in. I'll explain how we work things around here!"

The moment of truth had arrived. I walked back to the bleachers, set my towel down next to Wayne's, and stripped down to my swimsuit. Then I dashed back to the lane and quickly got in.

Joan explained the drills and how we shared the lane; then we started swimming.

It was tiring, but invigorating. Joan couldn't have been nicer. Before I knew it, practice was over and everyone was getting out. Wayne came over to check on me.

"How'd you do? It looks like you survived."

"I'm still afloat," I reassured him.

"You hungry? Some of the team is grabbing a bite after. Want to join them?"

"I don't know…"

"You should go," Joan encouraged. "I have to get home. But I think they're going to Pizza Palace. Have you been yet?"

I shook my head.

"It's really good Italian food. You'd have fun. Great way to get to know everyone," she said.

"If you want to go, I guess that'd be fine," I said to Wayne.

"Great!" he said. "But… that means you'll have to get out of the water."

I looked toward my towel, A.K.A. my Thigh Shield. It was blocked by a gaggle of swimmers.

Wayne was right. There were all ages and body types present. The swim team wasn't comprised of the *Baywatch* hard body studs

> *My safety blanket (towel) was a few feet away, but it might as well have been miles.*

and beauties I had imagined. They were regular folks, some more toned than others, who were currently drying off and talking about everything from work and kids to swim strokes and current events.

How I envied them their casualness; they were in no hurry to hide their bodies.

The fact still remained that I was embarrassed about my body and I was about to expose it for all to see.

Hesitantly, I climbed out of the water and tried to rush to my towel as inconspicuously as possible. Before I got to it, someone shouted, "Hey, Wayne! Is that your wife?"

Suddenly, I was living a nightmare. Me. Dripping wet. Thighs totally exposed. The center of attention.

My safety blanket (towel) was a few feet away, but it might as well have been miles. There have been few times in life I have felt so exposed or vulnerable.

But everyone was so nice and welcoming. No one stared at my legs. No one gagged or threw up at the sight of them.

I look back on that now and laugh. Swim team was the best thing that ever happened to my body image. I never got ripped or lean from swimming. But I learned new skills, like flip turns and the butterfly stroke. And by the end of that summer I was standing around after practice talking and laughing without rushing to cover myself up anymore.

Because that was the best part of all — I made friends. Ones who accepted me as I am, warts and all. Or, in my case, cellulite thunder thighs and all.

~Courtney Lynn Mroch

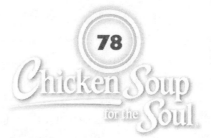

78

Sizing Up My Life

To accept ourselves as we are means to value our
imperfections as much as our perfections.
~Sandra Bierig

I went into the store with one intention — to upgrade my wardrobe. Not to a more expensive, name-brand label, but to the next size up. It was a big deal.

I was forty-five and had overcome an eating disorder. From age fourteen to my early twenties, I was anorexic and bulimic. It was what defined me. It was who I was.

During those years, being small, thin, and below a certain weight was my defense from rejection. I thought that if I couldn't be flawless, like my beauty queen friend, I could at least be perfectly thin.

Then I married, became a mom, and realized love wasn't dependent on how I looked. Though I didn't fixate as much on losing weight, I still tried to keep things under control by running several miles each week.

By forty-five, my life was too hectic to manage work and parenting and the rest of my life, and I cut down on the running. Gradually, I gained weight.

It was a big deal for me, not because it sent me back to disordered eating, but because I chose to handle it differently. Instead of loathing my body when my clothes were too tight and starving to lose weight, I decided to get clothes which I felt comfortable and confident in for my new phase of life.

So I went to an upscale resale shop and found the "medium" section.

And I tried on lots of clothes.

I spent two hours inside that dressing room, looking in the mirrors. Instead of seeing a woman I didn't want to be, I saw the reflection of someone who looked good in clothes that complemented her body.

For me, it was a first.

> *It was the first time I allowed myself to try on a different size.*

It was the first time I allowed myself to try on a different size. The first time I didn't wish to be smaller. The first time I chose to accept myself as I was and didn't fixate on trying to change my body.

I spent more money than I probably should have that afternoon. When I came home, I laid my purchases on the couch. Before my husband made any comments about money or asked if I really needed what I bought, I looked him in the eye and asked for his attention.

"Honey," I said, "I need you to listen." With tears in my eyes, I told him what I bought and simply said, "This is a big deal. I am tired of not liking who I am when my clothes don't fit. I want to feel good with how I am now. This was really hard for me."

He looked at me and smiled. He asked me to model the purchases and give him a fashion show. He never asked how much I spent or what I was going to do with the too-small clothes in my closet.

He gave me the gift I had just given myself — acceptance of a body that years ago I would have rejected.

And the gift to be okay with who I am now.

It was a big deal.

~Brenda Lazzaro Yoder

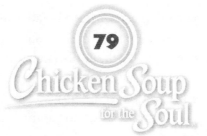

The Weight of Laughter

I finally realized that being grateful to my body was
key to giving more love to myself.
~Oprah Winfrey, O The Oprah Magazine

I overcame my eating disorder five years ago. Since then, I have avoided scales. At regular doctor checkups, I would close my eyes or gaze at the ceiling when I got weighed.

I ate healthy, hiked often, and indulged in foods I loved. On the outside I was completely recovered. But secretly, I still feared the scale. I feared its power over me, and its crippling ability to steal my desire to eat. I feared who I would become if I knew how much I weighed. I feared my husband would no longer be proud of my strength and determination if I got upset about a number.

I bought a scale. I wanted to keep it a secret, hidden under our bed, but I knew I had to tell him. Our marriage is based on trust, and that little purposeful lie of omission would gnaw at me. I had to tell him to keep myself accountable.

But lately I felt stronger. I felt curious about my new body, with its strong muscles and soft edges. I felt as though weighing myself might destroy the last barriers of my eating disorder, despite the risk of sending myself spiraling into a black hole of despair. I needed to know how much I weighed to accept myself. It was a way to prove my recovery — the harshest test of all.

I stripped off my clothes and prepared to step onto the scale. After all, every cotton fiber adds up and the old habit lingered.

I closed my eyes and heaved a deep breath through my nose and out my mouth. I stepped onto the scale. My stomach rolled. I opened my eyes, and registered the black numbers glaring up at me.

I laughed. It was not a hysterical laugh, the type that gurgles from my throat, making me feel oxygen-deprived. It was a laugh of pure joy. I was staring at the heaviest weight I had ever seen, and I was surprisingly okay with it.

> *I gained 20 pounds and still my husband loved me and kissed me and gazed at me in awe.*

The immense relief stemmed from living years defined by a number.

I had gained 20 pounds, and still I could read, write, jump, and play. I gained 20 pounds and still my husband loved me and kissed me and gazed at me in awe. Twenty pounds and still I hiked mountains. Twenty pounds and still I painted Disney characters, savored ice cream, rode horses, and laughed with friends. Twenty pounds and my life was not over. In fact, it was more joyful than ever, probably on account of the ice cream.

I stepped off the scale, contemplating my newfound freedom. Free from fear of a number, free from fear of a relapse. I felt healed and whole.

The number did not define me that morning, and it never will again.

~Shelby Kisgen

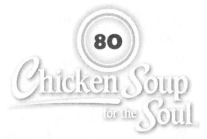

80

SweetestRedHead

As if you were on fire from within. The moon
lives in the lining of your skin.
~Pablo Neruda, Ode to a Beautiful Nude

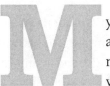

y last divorce had devastated my psyche. I found a dating site, although I was fearful of something new. I felt like a broken down old man. Who would want me at fifty-five?

A confident and curvy lady nicknamed SweetestRedHead accidentally clicked on my profile, still lacking a photo. Even more accidental was the automatic flirt she sent while trying to exit my profile, asking for a photo. I hesitantly took the worst selfie in the world and submitted it. I was many pounds overweight and hurting both physically and emotionally.

With no confidence I wrote back to this lady. She wrote back. Said I was handsome. How could this beautiful creature, this SweetestRedHead, see that in me? We continued on, e-mail after e-mail, one self-revelation after another. It was actually exciting to come home from work to see her next e-mails. She felt the same. I finally got up the nerve to ask her out! A date was set for Friday, 6:45 P.M.

I was early to the restaurant by nearly an hour. I waited outside. As she walked up, I knew it was her. I could tell by her photos that she was curvy but this was more than I expected. But, because of our e-mails, I was still so excited to meet her in person. Dinner was wonderful. She eventually invited me to sit next to her. I wondered if she could hear the beating of my heart. A soft touch and we held hands. No words needed to be spoken but many were said. When we finally looked up, after hours of conversation, the place was cleared of other patrons. The workers were eating their post-shift meal and waved at us genially as we left. Word had gotten around about our "blind date" and they left us two lovebirds alone.

I walked her to the car and we hugged goodbye. I could feel the tensions in my body release from her heartfelt embrace. I kissed her gently, sensing her surprise. She was not that kind of girl. My kiss so tender did something for her. She kissed back with her own tenderness evident. We broke apart with reluctance as she got in her car and drove away. I watched her car till it was no longer visible. We both drove home all agog. Whatever just happened was incredible! We needed more of each other.

Our romance was a whirlwind. She, ever so confident in her curves hidden by clothes, became hesitant when it was time to become intimate. I examined her curves with the one thing I had going for me, my absolute adoration of her. I showed it with my eyes. She was inexperienced and often hesitant. My patience was rewarded with her acceptance.

In the glow after, she nestled into my side. Being the poker player I am, I sensed her "tell" — that she wondered if she was worthy. I never told her what her tell was. It was an ever so slight unconscious nodding of her head. Happened almost every time, especially while snuggling together. I would tease her about it, but never revealed it. Looking into her adoring eyes and seeing that adoration being returned soon eased her "tell" and led us to a beautiful life together.

I could see, when she looked at me, how loved I was. She could see, when I looked at her, how loved she was. Our confidence in ourselves soared and that in turn fed our love. She found she didn't have to hide the curves of a beautiful woman. She didn't have to feel uneasy about nudity. What did I see after all? I saw a woman who loved me so much that my heart yearned for her every minute we were apart. I saw a woman whose being filled my soul. I saw a woman who filled my confidence with just a loving look from her soft brown eyes. I was no longer the broken down old man she rescued like a puppy from the pound. I was vibrant and strong. I had confidence again. I was whole and we were united in our love.

She had been alone most of her adult life. Caring full-time for an aging and ailing parent left little room for others. Four years before meeting me, her mother had passed away. Her friends I met told me how happy I'd made her. They just didn't get it. I had to tell them how happy she made me! I would have shouted it from the rooftops!

We promised each other forty years together. We cooked together, cleaned and took the garbage out as one. A team, synchronized. When I had to go on the occasional trip, we e-mailed or texted constantly. I filled her in on my days as I traveled for work, announcing my next location. I would text my ETA for arriving home, sometimes beating traffic. Her joy at seeing me, and my joy in seeing her, fed us like a food. We craved each other, unable to be sated. We encouraged each other for work and play.

Our confidence in ourselves soared and that in turn fed our love. She found she didn't have to hide the curves of a beautiful woman.

Then, some discomfort. A doctor visit. More painful visits. I skipped work to be with her at every appointment. Then a visit to a specialist an hour away. Several weeks later we were back and a surgeon's skills were used. That was followed by a day in the hospital. I slept on a chair in her room. Next, ten weeks of recovery. No lifting, cooking, cleaning. I was nursemaid, cook, and assistant all rolled into one. I gave it my best effort.

My beautiful, curvy, and adored SweetestRedHead passed away before any additional treatment could be done. The paramedics were heroic as I sat stunned at what was happening.

We didn't get forty years. We had two and a half. Best years of my life. God had other plans for her. God has plans for me too and I will accept his call when my time comes. She would want me to be happy. I know that. I was happy just being with her.

In heaven, they say you are perfect. Here on earth, she already was for me.

~Patrick Michael McIntyre

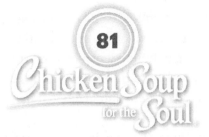

81

Hairpin and Dangerous

Once we believe in ourselves, we can risk curiosity,
wonder, spontaneous delight, or any experience that
reveals the human spirit.
~E. E. Cummings

My dark hair and green eyes have always been my most noticeable features. I've had a lot of compliments on my "porcelain complexion" and been told I had "a pretty face." People have often felt it necessary to comment on the parts of me not associated with my plus-size body.

"Body." The very word always felt foreign in my mouth, uncomfortable and full. My body was a cage, a prison, attached to my soul like a decades-long ball and chain.

In high school, I was heavier than my peers and was teased and ridiculed for it. I was fit, but 170 pounds and short, so I struggled to find stylish outfits for a teenager. My friends shopped for big name designers at the mall while I browsed the Women's section in department stores. I didn't realize at the time that the mainstream fashion industry offered few options for young, plus-sized women like myself. I just thought there was something wrong with me.

In college, clothing mattered significantly less. I spent late nights studying and early mornings trudging to class in oversized sweatshirts. Even pajama pants were acceptable for lounging in the dining hall and in the dorms.

The people I met in college cared more about my thoughts, ideas, and personality than the brand or size of the jeans I wore. I do remember one roommate dieting to fit into a pair of size 0 Tommy Hilfiger jeans. Mouth agape, I said, "I have never heard of a size 0!" She informed me that even a size 00 existed, and I stared at her in disbelief as if she were a lunatic.

"You've never seen a 0 in a pair of pants before?" she asked.

"Only after the 2 in the pair I have on!" I said, with a laugh.

As a first-time teacher with a master's degree, my style morphed again. This time, my clothing selections had nothing to do with weight; they focused on professionalism. I had to dress my body for a real job. Back to the department stores I went, to the Women's section. Here was a familiar land — a land of clothes devoid of style, but they fit and made me look old enough to do the job. My comfy jeans and T-shirts went to the back of my closet, replaced by pantsuits and uncomfortable heels that made me look as graceful as a giraffe on stilts.

This style lasted through five years (not the heels, which only made it two days), one failed marriage, one baby, and several additional pounds.

Two years after my divorce, when I decided to start dating again, I had no idea what clothes to wear. So I decided I wouldn't dress my body; I would, instead, dress my soul.

I bought flowing bohemian blouses with interesting patterns and black leggings. I filled my closets with flats, chunky jewelry, scarves and bangle bracelets á la Stevie Nicks. And also, to feed my soul, I played my piano and went to poetry readings. After work, I was excited to get home and read. I started taking better care of my body, adopted a wholly vegetarian diet, and joined a gym to meet new people while staying active.

Dressing myself became effortless — but not because of the new items or a new body. My body was still my body and I was the heaviest I had ever been, tipping the scale at 250. I was still buying plus-sized clothes in the biggest sizes I had ever worn.

The difference was that now I was okay with that.

I had grown to live inside my body and truly inhabit it. It was mine — not just a hunk of flesh I was attached to as some sort of punishment. I was simply a plus-size woman; nothing more, nothing less.

A few years ago, I walked confidently into a bookstore where I was meeting a male friend from work to "talk shop." We had coffee and were checking out some short story collections to consider for classes. Half an hour into our great conversation, we were laughing in the magazine section together.

> *"I realized something I never noticed before. Your curves are hairpin and dangerous."*

"I can't stop thinking about kissing you," he suddenly said.

I was taken aback. Our meeting wasn't a date. But then, instead of being horrified, I was completely amused.

"Any particular reason?" I asked.

"I watched you walk from the bookshelves over to the coffee counter," he said, "and I realized something I never noticed before. Your curves are hairpin and dangerous."

Right there, in the middle of Books-a-Million, I kissed that man.

I didn't kiss him because he paid me a compliment or because it was a romantic thing to say or because I had thoughts about a relationship with him.

I kissed him as a celebration of the awareness that my body, after all these years, finally belonged to me.

And because as a beautiful, plus-size woman, I was able to tell it what to do without fear, regret, shame, or hurt — no matter what clothes I dressed it in.

~Stephanie Tolliver Hyman

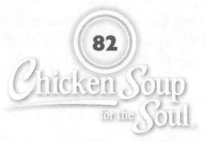

82

Holy Calves

When you're always trying to conform to the norm,
you lose your uniqueness, which can be the
foundation for your greatness.
~Dale Archer

My father was the first one to point out my unusually large leg muscles. I was just a gangly kid, maybe ten or eleven, and I'd never thought about the shape of my body before.

"You've got legs just like your mother," he said with a smile, ruffling my blond hair.

After he made that comment, I started scrutinizing other girls' legs and comparing them to my own. I could tell that my legs were different, and when you're a kid, being different is not a good thing.

I stood in front of the mirror and inspected my legs from every angle. From the front, my calf muscles jutted out so much that they joined together in the middle. From the side, they bulged out like baseball bats, hard and bulbous. From the back, they were inconceivably large. If I stood on my tippy toes, my calf muscles appeared thinner from the front, but even bigger from the back and side.

My leg muscles were enormous no matter which way I turned. Why couldn't I just have stick straight legs like the other girls in my class?

To top it all off, my mother wouldn't let me shave them. To put it simply, I had man legs. What had I ever done to deserve such muscular legs? I had the body of a pro athlete, but besides a few stints of soccer and swimming, I wasn't all that athletic.

Middle school gym class was the worst part of my week. Sitting beside the cool girls on the bleachers, waiting for my turn to run laps or shoot hoops, I was sure they were all staring at my mannish legs. I tried desperately to cover them by pulling my shorts as far down my thighs as possible, but this did little to hide my hairy secret. I was sure they were gawking at my ginormous calves.

Even on the hottest Florida days, I hid my bulky lower body beneath sweatpants and jeans. I gathered that men liked girls with petite bodies, and my monstrous legs made me anything but petite. I wanted to be feminine and delicate like the cool girls I admired in the halls. I watched the way the guys flirted with them, pinching their tiny waists playfully and slinging their arms over their thin, girlish shoulders.

I did everything I could to be like them. I wore ribbons in my hair like they did, making sure the color matched my outfit. I bought the chunkiest platform shoes I could find at the discount shoe store. I made my sister straighten the curls out of my hair with a clothing iron, kneeling beside the ironing board as she passed the hot metal as close to my scalp as possible. But I could never be like those girls with perfect, stick-straight bodies — not with my legs of steel.

One New Year's Eve, when I was midway through high school, my older cousin Maria stopped me on my way to the buffet table.

"Holy calves!" she said, pulling on my arm and turning me around. "Girl, you've got amazing legs."

"What?" I said, flustered, pulling down the hem of my knee-length dress.

"Seriously," she continued, flashing me a big smile. "I know so many people — girls and guys — who would kill for legs like that."

"Really?" I asked.

"Oh yeah! People do all kinds of crazy exercises to get legs as sculpted as yours. Leg lifts and squats and what not. And believe me," she said, leaning forward and lowering her voice. "Guys love girls with strong legs."

I let out a creaky laugh and slid out of her grasp. *She can't be serious,* I thought. But as she walked away, I noticed her legs beneath her tight skirt. She didn't have stick straight legs, either, but they didn't look terrible in a pair of high heels. Maybe there was some truth in her words.

After that, my idea about what a beautiful body looked like began to change. Instead of unconsciously consuming what glossy magazines showed me about beauty and femininity, I investigated my own feelings about the female body. Whoever said that being strong wasn't beautiful? I became less self-conscious about wearing shorts and skirts. So what if my legs were more muscular than those of your average football player? I decided there were more important things to worry about than the size of my calf muscles.

> *It is my hope that my children will grow up in a world that celebrates the beauty in women's strength.*

Over the years, my tolerance for these strong and curvy legs of mine turned to affection. People still stop their cars to comment on my muscular limbs when I'm strolling in my neighborhood, but I don't see the attention as negative anymore.

Once I realized all the amazing things that my strong legs allow me to do, I stopped wishing for my muscles to disappear. These legs have carried me many miles, across mountains and rough terrain. With my muscular legs, I can swim across lakes, pedal across continents, and dance until morning.

I'll never have the lithe build of the cool girls I looked up to in middle school, and there are some outfits that I cannot pull off because of my bulky frame. Some men might be intimidated by a woman with a body like mine, sculpted and strong, but those are not the men I am interested in. I can't change the fact that I was born with a muscular body, nor do I want to.

Instead, I have decided to lean into my body type. These days, I never think twice about wearing a pair of shorts, a tight skirt, or a short dress. In fact, the shorter the better.

I am no longer afraid of appearing strong, nor do I associate strength with manliness. It is my hope that my children will grow up in a world that celebrates the beauty in women's strength. My curvy legs are one of my many strengths, and I love showing them off to the world.

~Carmella de los Angeles Guiol

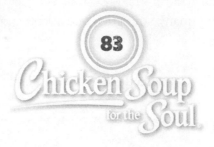
Skinny Dipping

And the day came when the risk to remain tight in a
bud was more painful than the risk it took to blossom.
~Anaïs Nin

"Come on, Mom! Get in the pool!" my five-year-old called from the water.

"Maybe a little later!" I said, with a forced smile, knowing full well I had just lied to my son. I sat in the shade of a patio umbrella, awash in guilt.

I really wanted to join him and splash with reckless abandon in the cool water. I wanted to hold him on my lap and careen down the water slide together, give him dolphin rides, and teach him how to float on his back. Instead, I sat on the deck and told him to stay in the shallow end.

Three things kept me rooted in that chair, baking in the hot sun. First was the space between my pool chair and the edge of the pool. Ten steps, to be precise. Ten steps to walk with no towel covering parts of me that my swimsuit wouldn't. Ten steps, feeling very much like a brontosaurus lumbering across the ground, legs jiggling for all to see. Ten steps might as well have been a mile.

Second, there were lots of people around. And not just any people. Family. At that moment I gladly would've traded my loved ones for a group of random strangers who would glance at me once and get back to their own business. Sharing an afternoon with family was so much worse. Strangers might silently judge the plus-size mom, but family will say it out loud, discuss it over coffee, and revisit the topic at regular intervals.

In particular, I was stressed over one very thin family member who wouldn't know what cellulite was if it came up to her and introduced itself. She had this rather predictable habit of coming up to me, giving my body a quick once-over, and then saying, "So… think you'll have any more kids?"

Lastly, and worst of all, the thing that kept me from jumping in the pool was myself. My own insecurities and expectations of what a bathing suit should look like on my body. Irrational thoughts about whether or not people would still like me if they saw what I really looked like, as if they couldn't already know my size from when I wore regular clothes.

A bead of sweat trickled down my back as the day grew warmer. I sat and watched my kids play with their cousins. I watched my brothers enjoy a rambunctious game of water basketball, and my mom swim with her grandkids. I watched my oldest sister take my son down the water slide, laughing joyfully, even though she has a shape much like mine. I was angry with myself for sitting on the sidelines of life and letting my weight stop me from living as fully as I should.

After a while, every part of me screamed for cool relief beneath the bright blue water. I rolled my pants up past my knees and sat at the edge of the pool. I'm sure I looked ridiculous sitting there in jeans and a T-shirt, but it was the best I could manage. The water on my calves was heaven. My brother-in-law noticed me sitting there. He swam over and hauled himself out of the pool. I half hoped he had come over to push me in, but instead he sat down next to me.

"Deb, why aren't you swimming?" he asked, with no hint of judgment in his voice.

I sat there for a minute and thought of all the reasons. My mind shuffled through one excuse after another until I sighed and said, "I just can't. I feel so fat."

"Well, let me ask you this," he said. "If you were here all alone, and there was no one else to see you, would you put on a suit and get in the pool?"

I burst out laughing and said, "If I were all alone, I'd be going down that slide stark naked!"

> *I dropped my towel on a chair. Left my insecurities there, too.*

He smiled and shrugged as if to say, "Then what are you waiting for?"

I had to admit, the man made an excellent point. He jumped back in and swam away and I went inside and changed. I nearly lost my nerve as I approached the pool, towel clutched tight against me.

But at that moment my son saw me standing there and his eyes lit up.

"Mom!" he screamed loud enough for the entire neighborhood to hear. "Mom's getting in the pool!"

What else could I do? I dropped my towel on a chair. Left my insecurities there, too. And I got in the pool.

~Debra Mayhew

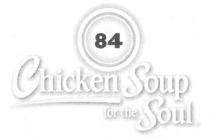

84

My Mom Called Me Sexy and I Agree

*If we all did the things we are capable of doing, we
would literally astound ourselves.*
~Thomas Edison

My seventy-three-year-old, stroke-surviving, cancer-surviving mom called me sexy as I walked into her hospital room, and it felt damn good.

I laughed as soon as I heard it. She laughed, too. We hugged and kissed, and then I took a seat on an uncomfortable chair in her room — feeling sexy as ever.

Do you know what I had on? Shorts, flip-flops, and a tank top. Nothing fancy. Just something I threw on so I could get things done that day. But do you know what made my mom call me sexy? My confidence. My head held high, the stride in my steps, the smile on my face.

When my mom saw all of that, she realized that I was comfortable in my own skin. I know that realization made her happy. It makes me happy, too.

This road to self-love hasn't been easy. As a matter of fact, it's been downright hard. Exhausting. Discouraging at times. But here I stand, after thirty-seven years on this earth, and I feel good about who I am, what I look like, and how I show up in the world. I make no apologies for the way that I laugh, the size of my feet, or the junk in my trunk.

I've never been thin. Even when I lost more than 40 pounds in my early twenties and my aunt affectionately referred to me as "skinny mini," I was still a size 8 or 10. Skinny in my opinion, but not thin enough by some standards. Still, I was happy with the weight loss. I felt good about life.

At just twenty-one years old, I was already familiar with the burden that comes with yo-yo dieting. I tried dieting teas. I joined the gym when we really couldn't afford it. I ate salads. I tried to avoid eating altogether (that never worked for more than a day). My choices were damaging to say the least. And all I wanted was to feel comfortable in my skin.

There wasn't a magic number or size. I simply wanted to love my body.

But losing weight didn't result in lasting confidence. Gaining it back after having two kids definitely didn't help. The only thing that helped me was having a few deep conversations with God and myself, developing an understanding about what life is really all about.

And now, I get it. I love the woman I've become, and I am so grateful my mom sees that. I have a daughter. She's only three, but I pray that as she gets older, she sees it too. I want her to realize that apologizing for who you are is no way to live. I want her to ignore anyone who has the nerve to make her think she isn't good enough.

So how do I walk in all this confidence, proud of my hips and thighs? I work at it. Every single day. It's hard work.

I work out most days of the week. Not because I want to be a size 6, but because I want to live. After giving birth to two kids, I see, with a new set of lenses, how important it is for me to live. After watching my mother suffer a stroke, depression, falls, cancer, and so much more, I see what my future could look like if my health fails.

I don't want that for myself. I don't want that for my kids.

And to be honest with you, the notion of feeling bad about a body that was strong enough to complete a marathon and then go on to give birth years later is just stupid.

My advice is simple: Tap into your strength. Think about all the things your body has done for you. All the experiences you've had.

All the trials you've endured. All the people who love you just the way you are.

Then let those thoughts stay with you. Always. Let those thoughts become a daily mantra. Let those thoughts take over.

> *Tap into your strength. Think about all the things your body has done for you.*

Thin doesn't equal healthy or happy. Healthy living equals healthy and happy. It's really that simple.

Pray. Go to therapy. Exercise. Sleep well. Say "no" with confidence. Say "yes" with enthusiasm. Spend time with people who lift you up. Have fun. Enjoy life.

My confidence is the root of my joy and that confidence doesn't come from what I look like. It comes from what I believe about myself.

~Martine L. Foreman

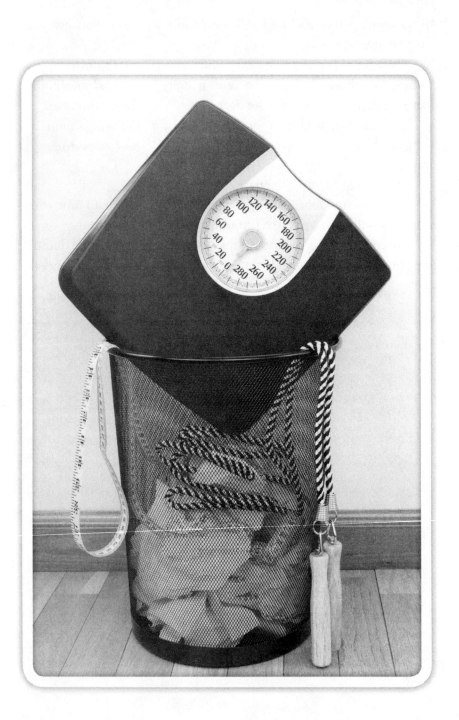

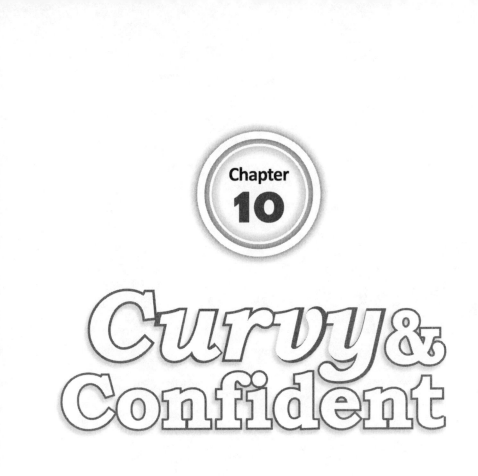

Chapter

10

Curvy & Confident

Breaking Out of
My Comfort Zone

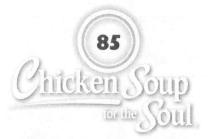

85

The Perfect Dress

*Just around the corner in every woman's mind — is a
lovely dress, a wonderful suit, or entire costume which
will make an enchanting new creature of her.*
~Wilhela Cushman

I was on a mission to find the perfect dress for my husband's graduation from pharmacy school. I had already tried on a few dresses and hadn't found "the one" yet, but this rack showed promise.

I enlisted my husband to help me search for my size. I pointed out the dresses I was interested in and gave him his instructions.

What I didn't disclose was my internal checklist: Would the fabric stretch to cover my broad shoulders? Did it look too fancy? Could I wear leggings under it so I didn't have to show my pale legs? Could I throw a cardigan or jean jacket over it to hide my flabby arms? Finally, the most important question: Would it hide enough of my flaws so that I would feel beautiful?

"What about this one?" my husband asked.

"That's pretty."

He was holding a sleeveless navy dress with a chevron-patterned skirt. It had a keyhole cutout at the neckline embellished with a silver piece just above it. The skirt looked about knee length. It was the type of dress meant to stand alone and make a statement.

But no cardigan or jacket would ever work with it. Leggings would be impossible. The dress didn't meet any of my secret criteria. I nearly told him it wouldn't work, but I decided to give him the benefit of the doubt. It was his graduation I'd be wearing it to after all, and he had proven to have good taste in the past.

I took the dress into the changing room with my other, more sensible choices just to appease him. I knew it wouldn't work, not with the amount of leg I'd be showing and that sleeveless top. But to my complete surprise, I liked it.

> *The dress didn't meet any of my secret criteria.*

The silver embellishment at the neckline wasn't too fancy for me after all. And though the skirt was shorter than what I usually wore, I realized I looked good in it. The dress was stunning and I couldn't help but feel beautiful in it, in spite of my pale legs and un-toned arms.

I stepped out of the dressing room to show my husband. The look on his face told me I'd found the perfect dress. Well, technically, *he* had found the perfect dress, despite breaking every fashion rule he didn't know I had. I walked out of the store that day with more than just a dress to wear to his graduation. I walked out with confidence I hadn't carried in with me, and without my secret checklist.

~Beth Pugh

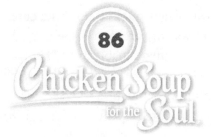

86

Yoga. Brunch.

*Yoga has a sly, clever way of short-circuiting the
mental patterns that cause anxiety.*
~Baxter Bell, MD

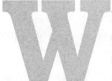hen had I become so weak? I mean honestly. I
don't mean to start this story off with such a self-
deprecating question, but it sure is a legitimate
one.

I used to be so confident. Maybe it was when friends and family
started making comments about my new size 20 body. Sure, I had
been a bangin' size 4 not too long ago, but I was still me. And Me was
still pretty great... right?

When had I started feeling bad for myself? Not wearing make-up?
Not buying cute clothes? Not caring an ounce about what I looked
like? When had I started to allow others' opinions to stunt my social
life? I no longer went out because it was hard for me to walk. I got
tired easily. I couldn't stand looking in the mirror.

I chose the couch over a night out. And sweat pants over jeans,
because I didn't have a pair that fit. If I couldn't wear sweats, I wasn't
going. I loathed going to work because I was a prisoner to muumuu
dresses and tight slacks.

I was consumed by what people thought of me and scared of what
they might say. At what point was it that I started to care?

When had I become so weak?

That was all I thought about as I stared at my e-mail in horror. I was given a shot with a new publication about entertainment/nightlife. As a journalist, this was my dream job. Getting paid to drink, eat and live life was something unattainable a very short while ago, and now there it was, in my lap. All I had to do was impress the editor with my piece and everything was golden.

So why was I horrified by my trial assignment, you ask? Two words. Yoga. Brunch.

Okay. So the brunch part I could totally handle. But yoga. Really? My palms started to sweat and my eyes glazed over. I was not just out of shape, but I was wildly, WILDLY uncomfortable with my weight. I was nervous that I would be the biggest girl in the room, that people would be talking about me or that I wouldn't be able to complete the yoga session. I was nervous I would pass out. Or get sick. Or cry. Or all of the above. Of all the events in the city, this is the one I was assigned. Quite possibly the only workout-related event EVER.

But I really lusted after this job. Finally, I was given an opportunity, so I was determined not to blow it.

I just had to prepare myself properly. New clothing and a great night's sleep would help me master this challenge. I was sure of it.

As my husband and I walked through the clothing store I started to become even more uncomfortable. So many cute things that I would have looked so great in before. Back when I thought I was "fat." Wow, what I wouldn't give for that body today.

Yoga pants. I was confronted with a large towering shelf of cheap five-dollar pants. Different materials, different lengths, different daunting levels of tightness. I decided on the green label ones. They were the loosest I could find. But, like always, it appeared that the store was out of my size. Not many stores carried my size anymore, so I was already scraping the bottom of the barrel. But there, at the very tip top of the shelf was one last pair of size 2x yoga pants.

On to the sports bras. If shopping for workout clothes could get any worse this was going to be it. Finding sports bras that fit nicely was worse than trying to find real bras, which was actually worse than trying to find a nice bathing suit. I have always had big boobs. Always. And until recently it has been a blessing. No matter what size sports bras I chose the girls always seemed smushed into one big uni-boob. Half in. Half out. It's a tragic sight.

I chose the only 3x I could find. It was boring. Cotton. Stretchy. Yuck. Then I saw some more attractive ones that were bright pink and looked like actual sports bras instead of the boring piece of cloth I already had in my cart. "Go big or go home," I thought (no pun intended). I switched out the 3x boring bra for the fancy pants 2x bra, crossed my fingers and hoped for the best. I figured trying the clothing on in the fitting room would stress me out even more, so, deciding to just take a chance, we made our way to the register.

> *I tried desperately to wriggle my way out of this tiny torture device, but to no avail.*

On the way we passed some loose fitting, very trendy, workout tank tops.

Those would definitely hide my rolls!

I skimmed through the racks of funny sayings, and as chance would have it, the only one in my size was a tank with the words "Can you keep up?" The irony… Yes… Yes, they can.

Thinking it would be humorous, I added the shirt to my cart. I really wanted this job. And if I wasn't going to allow myself to cry, at least I would be able to laugh.

And laugh we did. Once home, I attempted to try on my new threads, but the shirt I purchased didn't have a full back. That's right. There was a huge slit, exposing all the fun parts of my very large backside. #Return.

Then for the sports bra. Turns out the fancy bra was not the wise choice after all.

I think just about every woman has had a run-in of some sort with a sports bra at least once in her life. Over the head. The straps get tangled. Your arms aren't long enough to pull the back part down.

I twisted and turned. Grunted and winced. Breaking a sweat, I slumped to the couch in utter defeat. Sports bra 1–Jamie 0. I tried desperately to wriggle my way out of this tiny torture device, but to no avail. Reinforcements would have to be called in. I would have to ask my husband for help.

Just as I was playing the scenario out in my head he wandered in to the room, took one look at me sprawled out on the couch with sweaty, grimy parts hanging out everywhere, and started laughing maniacally. Reaching down, as if I were a little girl who needed help getting dressed, he tried to pull down the front of the sports bra, but it wouldn't budge. At that point we were both laughing so hard tears streamed down our cheeks.

The yoga pants fit, and went on without incident, which was a confidence booster at that point. I chose a charity marathon T-shirt to wear (as if I had ever run a marathon in my life), but it would cover any body issues I had, so I was satisfied.

I laid out my new yoga pants, T-shirt and shoes, packed a bottle of water and placed my yoga mat by the door.

I couldn't sleep. The suspense was too much for me. The idea of yoga, in an ultra trendy part of town, early in the morning, while writing for a new publication, terrified me to the core, and my husband could tell. He rolled over, looked into my eyes and spoke the biggest truth.

"Don't forget, you define the moment. Don't let the moment define you," he said.

And he was right.

The morning came quickly. 8 A.M. on a Sunday. Yay. But I was determined. Plus, brunch and drinks were involved, so it could be worse.

After putting on my big girl panties, literally, I headed out the door.

And ya know what? It ended up being okay.

I was the biggest girl there.

I was one of the only ones who didn't complete all the poses. But I honored my body and did what I could.

I defined my moment and made a change in my life. I changed the way I viewed myself. I changed the way I approached my moments, and in that moment I made the choice to change my life.

Namaste.

~Jamie Leigh Miller

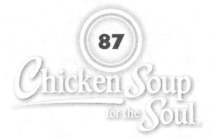

Picture Perfect

You have been criticizing yourself for years, and
it hasn't worked. Try approving of yourself
and see what happens.
~Louise L. Hay

lick! I whipped my head around. My husband was taking another candid photo of me with his cell phone.

That click was my nemesis. I never seemed to hear it when I felt my cutest.

"Look at this!" he'd exclaim. My husband loved every photo. I hated them. Where he saw beauty, I only saw flaws. When did my butt become so large? Why was I so flat chested? Was that stubble on my legs?

I feared that the photos would somehow escape into "the cloud," to be seen by friends and co-workers, or worse, turn up on my daughter's iPad to traumatize her childhood.

I demanded he delete the latest photo. He was heartbroken. And that's when I felt guilty. He meant well. He was just being playful and he truly loved the photos. Here he was, finding me attractive, and I was chastising him for it.

I got tired of this pattern, and one day, through sheer exasperation — and a touch of insanity — I decided to take matters into my own hands. If my hubby wanted pictures, I would give him pictures. I booked a photo session with a boudoir photographer.

It was absolutely terrifying, but if I could get through the photo session I could surprise my husband with the photos. And then maybe he'd stop taking all those candid shots when I was not exactly at my best.

By the time I reached the studio my heart was racing. I took a few deep breaths to calm myself.

I wanted to do this.

I needed to do this.

I needed to face my insecurity.

With a CD of my favorite music in hand and my "armor" of professional hair and make-up, I stepped into the studio and introduced myself to the photographer.

> *If my hubby wanted pictures, I would give him pictures. I booked a photo session with a boudoir photographer.*

I had spent hours searching for the right photographer and as soon as I saw Dario's photographs, I knew he was the one. His photographs were works of art. One image in particular resonated with me. It showed a woman standing in front of a mirror applying lipstick; her stomach was bare and it was obvious she had carried a child. Any modern magazine would have retouched the photograph, smoothing out her stomach to perfection. In Dario's photo her stomach was left untouched and it was beautiful.

I spent the afternoon having photograph after photograph taken. For years I had compared myself to the glossy images in my favorite fashion magazines. I knew the photos were carefully orchestrated but I had no idea how much went into creating the perfect photograph until I experienced it myself. The lighting, the props, the hair, the clothing, the slightest adjustment to how my body was positioned — each was essential to creating a "casual" photograph. By the end of the day, I was utterly exhausted and my muscles ached. I left the studio with a new understanding for what went into the "perfect" images I often resented seeing in magazines.

I had booked the boudoir photo session to create a gift for my husband. What I didn't expect was a gift for myself. I spent a day feeling entirely vulnerable as I faced all of my insecurities about my body head on. Yet, as I looked through the photographs that resulted from that session I saw my body in a way I had never seen it before. I didn't see a large butt. Instead, I saw the sexy way my back dipped just above it. I didn't see leg stubble. Instead, I saw beautifully shaped calves I didn't even realize I had. I didn't see a flat chest. Instead, I saw a body proportioned exactly as it should be.

I saw a woman finally confident in her own skin. I saw me.

~Robin R.

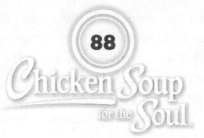

Twenty-Dollar Muse

I've never felt more beautiful or more
like myself... I love my body.
~Amy Schumer after shooting
the Pirelli 2016 Calendar

I'd always known I was beautiful. I had an hourglass figure and wore a 34C bra. Then I got to college. I loved my liberal arts college, but it was stressful. To comfort the stress, there was the cafeteria. And the bistro. And the convenience store.

The Freshman Fifteen wasn't bad, but it turned into the Sophomore Forty. I didn't notice it happening; because I was beautiful, I rarely looked in the mirror. One day my best friend, Dana, took me to her full-length mirror and said, "It's time to start dressing the body you have, not the body you want."

I looked and saw everything. The bulging thighs. The sagging butt. The stretch lines. The drooping breasts. Dana had always been plus-sized and always looked amazing. She told me she'd take me shopping and show me her tricks.

But going shopping required money, and I hadn't had a job in over a year.

I took a job in a mailroom working the sunrise shift — 5:45 A.M. until 9 A.M., skipping breakfast and attending a full day of classes on very little sleep. Less than four hours a day, five days a week, at minimum wage. I made less than $20 in the first week and quit by Saturday.

My friend Jason, an art major, had an idea. I posed for him so he could practice his drawing, for which he paid me $10 for two hours. As I was leaving, he said: "You'd do great as an art model. I can get you in, if you're ever interested."

Art modeling — a glamorous term for getting naked in front of strangers, letting them stare at you and doodle, I thought to myself.

"It's $20 an hour," Jason added.

I needed bras that didn't squeeze my back and leave red marks under my breasts. I needed shirts that didn't look like they were going to pop their buttons. Even if I shopped at Goodwill, I would need some money. *I was at a liberal arts college, there to learn about myself and to try new things.* Also, it was $20 an hour. Sometimes sessions lasted five hours, he said, and $100 was nothing to sniff at.

My first day, I wore my good clothes — it shouldn't have mattered since I was there to take them off, but I wanted to look nice. The teacher, Mr. Godfrey, a little old man with glasses that slipped down his nose, gently shook my hand and showed me to a tiny dressing room with a fluffy robe waiting for me. When I came back, wrapped in my long robe, I surveyed the room. It was a softly lit room with small tables arranged around a raised platform. Not easels, Mr. Godfrey explained, because it was a sculpture class. I'd pose on a platform, which turned like a lazy Susan, and relax. From time to time, a student would turn the platform, but that wasn't for me to worry about.

The students hadn't come in yet, so I tried the platform — hard wood. I frowned, and Mr. Godfrey immediately brought over some pillows. "We want you to be comfortable," he smiled. "You're our muse."

Students filtered in and I clutched my robe closer, perched on the pillows. They chatted with their friends about the movie shown the previous night — *The Matrix.* There were about ten of them. I'd expected a huge, anonymous auditorium with nameless faces. I didn't know their names, but they weren't strangers — I'd seen them before, in passing on the way to psych class or sipping coffee in the cafeteria.

Mr. Godfrey greeted the class and explained a few things about working with clay, capturing the natural form, and other technical terms I didn't understand. He ended by saying, "Everyone, meet Lauren."

Breaking Out of My Comfort Zone |

The class applauded loudly. Mr. Godfrey smiled his grandfatherly smile at me. "Shall we begin?"

I slowly let the robe fall from my shoulders, past my wide hips, and collapse in a pile around my ankles. "Get comfortable," said Mr. Godfrey. I tried to gracefully sit on the pillows, but I floundered around them, finally just lying on my back and throwing my limbs around like a rag doll. I couldn't see the students, just the stained ceiling and the vent system. I could feel the cold air blow down my breasts and across my thighs.

Mr. Godfrey said, "You must be cold, dearie," and set up a space heater next to me. I felt the rush of hot air relax my muscles and I settled back further into the pillows. I heard a click and soft, classical piano music filled the air.

> "You're pure art," he smiled. "We can't create without you."

It was a peaceful place. I was warm, there was soothing music, and I was staring into space. Every now and then, someone walked up and gently turned my table a few degrees. I took breaks every thirty minutes or so, slipped the robe back on and walked around, looking at the clay replicas in various states of accuracy. Some were grotesque, some distorted, but the good ones, the ones with real form and clean lines, were beautiful. The students wandered around, commenting quietly on each other's work. I heard a few words — Rodin, Venus de Milo, Botticelli.

The hours passed quickly. As I pulled the robe on for the last time and the students packed up, one approached me. He had black and blue hair and honest eyes. "You were amazing," he said. "Really inspiring."

"Inspiring?" I cocked an eyebrow.

"You're pure art," he smiled. "We can't create without you." He adjusted his backpack, said, "See you," and left.

Mr. Godfrey turned off the heater and started counting out twenty-dollar bills. "The students loved you. You're a classic figure, like one of the Graces. I'd love to have you back next week." He handed me the money.

I didn't look at the cash in my hand. An unbidden smile spread across my cheeks and into my eyes. "I'd love to."

I kept modeling all through college and even for a few years after. It took getting naked in front of some college kids for me to first realize how beautiful I was. I don't know what happened to the art or the artists, but I do know that someday, down the road, a museum or a mom looked at an image of my body and said, "That is beautiful."

~Lauren B. H. Rossato

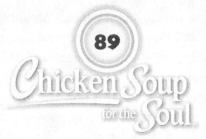

89

My Reflection in the Mirror

In your own life it's important to know
how spectacular you are.
~Steve Maraboli

I stared at my reflection in the full-length mirror for what seemed an eternity. Next to me were the dozens of dresses I'd already tossed into the "reject" pile.

Dress shopping for my thirty-year high school reunion had become very frustrating. I'd gained weight slowly over the years and wasn't used to my new large bosom and tummy pouch.

How could I possibly find a dress that looked good on me and how could I attend the reunion looking like this? I hadn't seen most of my classmates since high school graduation. Surely, everyone would notice I had gained weight. I felt embarrassed and ashamed. I finally settled on a simple black dress, one size too big, so it would be loose and cover my curves.

That evening I tried on the dress again at home. Who was I kidding? The dress looked horrible! Just then, as if on cue, my husband and young son walked in.

"Mom, what are you wearing?" My son giggled. "That dress is too big!"

My husband agreed. I looked at my reflection once more; I looked like I was wearing a sack. I don't know what came over me, but I started to laugh until happy tears fell. It felt so good to laugh! It must have been contagious, because we all stood there roaring with laughter.

I returned the dress the next day and in its place I bought a bright red, formfitting dress! This time when I stood in front of the mirror, I couldn't believe it — I loved what I saw.

"Wow, you're beautiful!" my husband said, when I twirled around to show him.

On the day of the reunion I was nervous. I timidly walked into the venue.

"Honey, there's no way you can't be seen with that beautiful red dress," my husband said. "Flaunt it!"

> *I returned the dress the next day and in its place I bought a bright red, formfitting dress!*

He knew just what to say to make me feel better, and he was right. Just then, one of my friends ran over to hug me.

"You look amazing," she said, excited. "I couldn't miss you walking in with that cute dress!"

That evening I reminisced, laughed and danced the night away.

That was nine years ago. Since then, I have learned to love my body and embrace my new curves instead of hiding them.

That moment I stood in front of the mirror was a turning point for me. I realized later that those dresses I tried on didn't look bad on my body; it was my insecurities that made them look bad.

My reflection in the mirror was the reflection of my lack of confidence. But nowadays, I love what I see!

~Dorann Weber

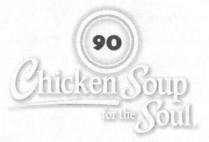

90

A Unique Vessel

Man is the sole animal whose nudity offends
his own companions, and the only one who,
in his natural actions, withdraws and
hides himself from his own kind.
~Michel de Montaigne

One summer morning, my husband said, "Hon, I know you've been taught being naked in public is perverted. The park's not like that. I wish you'd come with me to see for yourself. You don't have to undress. If you don't like it, I'll never ask again."

He was studying massage therapy and a few months earlier his instructor led a field trip to a naturist park. My husband loved it and wanted to go back.

I had been taught "flaunting" your body was morally wrong and I couldn't bring myself to go with him. Also, my body is deformed and I wasn't comfortable letting anyone see it naked.

But now, the more I thought about it, the more he made sense. I needed to find out for myself what really went on at the park, and if possible, I needed to be comfortable in my own skin. Maybe he was right. I agreed to go — reluctantly.

I have scoliosis, a curvature of the spine. I was eleven when my parents first noticed it. They had bought me a new dress with a tight bodice and flared skirt. I was twirling and laughing as the skirt swished against my legs until Mom stopped me. She called Dad to come and look at my back. "That zipper isn't straight. It's curving to one side."

"That's odd. Better have the doctor take a look."

We tried many different treatments but the curvature steadily increased. A hump, formed by my distended ribs, appeared on the left side of my back. My right shoulder drooped, and I had a peculiar gait. I felt like Quasimodo.

Eventually, I had a spinal fusion. This entailed removing bone from my leg and fusing the twelve inches of vertebrae between my neck and waist. I was fitted with a steel brace and had to attend rehab to learn to walk again.

On my first day back at school, I walked past a group of students standing by their lockers. "Hey, guys, look. We've got Igor with us this year."

They were laughing and pointing at me. I bolted from the building and ran home.

Every time I looked into the mirror, all I saw was the deformity. I thought I was ugly. A grey cloud of "not good enough" enveloped me.

The person who helped me accept myself was my husband. We had met when I was at the rehab home after my surgery, and three years later we married. I started to feel better about myself, but I still wasn't ready for anyone other than my husband to see my body.

But now we were on our way to a naturist park. "You know, we can turn around and go home. You don't have to do this," said my husband.

"No," I said. "I'll be okay. I'm scared, but I know you'll take me home if I don't like it."

At the entrance, I saw acres of rolling hills, forest and a small lake. Up the driveway stood a two-level building. To our right were buildings like motel units. Down the hill, I saw two teams playing volleyball amidst much laughter. All over the property, people were lounging in chairs reading, chatting and having fun. Others were swimming. It was like any joyful day at any large park — except that almost everyone was naked.

In the clubhouse we met the owners. They were naked. My face burned, but they smiled graciously and Barb took my hand in hers,

Breaking Out of My Comfort Zone |

saying, "Try not to be nervous. We've enjoyed having your husband here and we're glad you've decided to join him. Let's show you around. You don't have to take off any clothes. Naturism isn't for everyone and we want you to be comfortable."

After walking through the clubhouse, we strolled the environs. Everyone greeted us with a smile or a wave. I discovered I could look people in the eye and engage in conversation without being embarrassed. I saw whole families playing, swimming, barbequing and just relaxing in the sun. There wasn't anything "sexy" about it. No one was "flaunting" their shapely curves or six-pack abs. Most of the people were very ordinary—tall, short, thin, heavyset, elderly, young—just people out for a day in the sunshine.

It was like any joyful day at any large park—except that almost everyone was naked.

The owner explained to me that Naturism is a lifestyle that promotes a healthy body image and acceptance of your body. It's a way of life in harmony with nature that encourages a respect for self and others.

As the day wore on, I began to relax. I still wasn't ready to shed my own clothes but I did decide I could continue visiting.

After about two months, I could wear a long T-shirt there with nothing underneath. One very hot day, I looked longingly toward the lake. The park has a strict rule; no bathing suits or other clothing are allowed when swimming. Scanty bathing suits are enticing and emphasize much more sexiness than the naked body. If I wanted to go in the water, I had to take off my T-shirt.

With as much courage as I could muster, I stripped off my shirt, stood up tall and strode into the water. For the first time in my life, I was skinny-dipping! I couldn't believe how free I felt. The water slid off my arms like the finest silk. Every inch of me cooled and nothing constricted anywhere. I hooted with glee.

When I finally got out, longtime members smiled and nodded. Nobody cared that I was bent and crooked. Nobody cared that I didn't look like a model. They were all happy that I discovered for myself the joy of being sky-clad.

I have come to appreciate the unusual body I live in. I watch in wonder as it changes and ages. It feels good to stand on soft grass in the hush of the early morning clad in nothing but what the Creator gave me; or to take an outdoor shower and then dry off in the warmth of the sun without shame.

As different as my body is, I no longer define my self-worth by what I look like. I am so much more than "just a body." I am me, warts and all, privileged to live for a short time in this unique vessel.

~Maighread MacKay

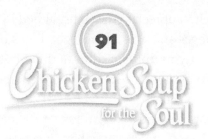

91

Mother of the Groom

You cannot be lonely if you like the
person you're alone with.
~Wayne W. Dyer

No dress. The wedding's a month away. My sister vetoed my first outfit as not suitable for the "Mother of the Groom." I've procrastinated, dreading shopping for an outfit that will beautify my plentiful curves. Not to mention the presence of my ex and his second wife's Barbie doll shape.

Thankfully, my Italian hairdresser suggests a small dress store owned by her cousin, insisting I call from her salon. A cheery, heavily accented voice greets my inquiry for a Mother of the Groom dress. "You come now. We fixa you." An offer I can't refuse.

Two old Italian ladies greet me. "Me owner," the smaller one claims. "Her, assistant," she points to a stout woman, a head taller. A flood of Italian begins as gnarly hands pat and pinch various parts of my body, turning me around as if selecting produce. Shock prevents me from vocalizing alarm. The private conference continues as the owner gestures toward a rack of gowns. Dresses are held in front of me as the rapid fire Italian bounces off the walls. No one asks my preferences. Unconsciously, I raise my hand. The women nod, ignoring my gesture. "My sister didn't like the first dress I chose," I state nervously.

Temporary ceasefire. "Sista no like?" one asks. "We finda one sista like," the other proclaims. The owner pushes me inside a dressing room. The assistant places three gowns on the hook. Apparently my vote doesn't count.

The first evening gown is rust-colored with a smock bodice. Opening the door, I gesture toward the back zipper. Expert hands turn me around, zipping me up. Sensing my wish to bolt, the stout woman's well-muscled arm leads me into the room to the center stage mirror. In unison, both crones shake their head no: "Nota good color."

"How will I zip my dress?" I wonder.

"Husband," they respond.

Raising my ring-less hand, I explain, "No husband. Divorce."

"Escort," they fire back.

"No escort," I clarify.

"No escort?" they ask, turning to each other shocked. Looking back at me, they say in unison, "Sista help you, Sista help you," their newly discovered mantra. Feelings of loneliness descend on me. Maybe I should rent an escort.

> *The smooth lines of the dress accent my curves, hiding my self-declared problem areas.*

Next is the navy gown with the high collar. It is met with shaking heads of dismay.

The last gown, a muted celery green, has a square neckline with embroidered gold straps. There's a jacket trimmed in matching gold embroidery. It looks elegant. Glancing at the price tag, I shudder. The assistant zips me up as I enter the room. They pace from my front to my back. Silence reigns. The women glance at each other, "Yes, yes, yes!" they say, clapping their hands. Their heads nod enthusiastically.

I glance into the mirrors again, shifting my body to view various angles. The smooth lines of the dress accent my curves, hiding my self-declared problem areas. I feel regal. Then I remember the price tag. "It's too expensive," I say — half my mortgage payment to be exact.

"You sit with *familia*?" the stout woman inquires, ignoring my concern.

"Actually I'm at the head table," I answer. Their heads pop up, jerked by an invisible string. "It's a different approach," I explain.

"Head table with a no escort?" the owner asks with a frown.

"My younger son will be with me. He's the best man. At the table will be my son the groom, future daughter-in-law, her parents, maid of honor and her date, my ex and his wife — "

"Stoppa!" shouts the owner. "Stoppa!" She raises her hands as if to ward off a blow.

"Ex's wife? No good."

"Yes," I confirm, looking forlorn as I add, "she's much younger than I."

"No, no, no," she replies. Another burst of Italian fills the air accompanied by frantic hand gestures. The muscled assistant grabs my elbow; the owner pushes me from behind as I'm marched back into the dressing room amid clucking tongues. I'm taken out of the jacket. The owner yanks down the front of the gown while the assistant rummages behind me. She returns, wrapping me with a full strapless corset stretching from my belly button to bust, cutting off my air supply. "Takea bra off," the owner directs.

I release my bra. Noncompliance is not an option. The assistant begins strapping me in as if it were a straitjacket. My breasts point skyward with a perkiness lacking in my adolescence. This torture chamber leaves me vulnerable to confessing all my sins in the hope of mercy. "I can't breathe," I complain.

"Like watch, clamps on, youa forget," the owner responds, tweaking my breast like she's milking a cow. "This one too small, "she announces. "You need help."

I'm beyond help.

"We fixa. No one matches," she states, gripping one of her enormous breasts. "This one a bigger," she proclaims, bouncing her right breast in her hand. Out of her pocket comes padding. She pins it on the outside of the corset. "No inside, willa itch," she states.

"Who will get me into this?" I'm sharing a hotel room with my younger son. Seeing me in this contraption could result in years of therapy. I envision myself knocking on hotel doors at midnight begging for release.

"Sista help. You a needa look good," the owner replies, as I'm zipped and assisted into the jacket. I'm led to the mirrors. "Look neck.

Good neck. Wear jewelry," she instructs. The shopkeeper continues pointing at various body parts as if it's an anatomy lesson.

"Let'sa see arms." The jacket's removed. "Gooda arms!" she cries, rubbing her hands up and down them. "No skin. No drip." She points to her assistant's sagging upper arms. "No weara jacket. Take off. Showa arms. Letsa see legs." Both she and the assistant pull up the gown. "Gooda legs!" she shouts, raising her fingers to her mouth, smacking a kiss toward the ceiling. "We shorten gown, no? Showa leg."

"I'm not looking for a date," I protest.

"You a needa look good!" she retorts, smacking her hands together as if she'd rather take a swipe at me. The stout woman nods her head in agreement like a bobble head doll.

Their positive rating of my attributes leaves me perplexed; I'm unaccustomed to conducting my personal inventory in such a manner. It's an adjustment to view my body's terrain with identifiable assets. Reality settles in. While softly fingering the smooth dress material, I say, "The dress is too expensive."

"This you dress. You no like?"

"Yes, I like. It's beautiful but costs too much."

"You dress," she repeats. "Take $150 off dress, $100 off alterations. Good buy."

The two ladies are staring at me with heads angled to the side, questioning my reason. "Looka nice," the shopkeeper says timidly. They both agree, nodding, pointing to the dress. They declare in unison, "Sista like."

Realization dawns. Why am I worried about what others think? My happiness isn't dependent on someone else's opinion.

"Yes, Sista like." I'm ready to fly solo.

"Sold!" I say, as they applaud.

~Anne Merrigan

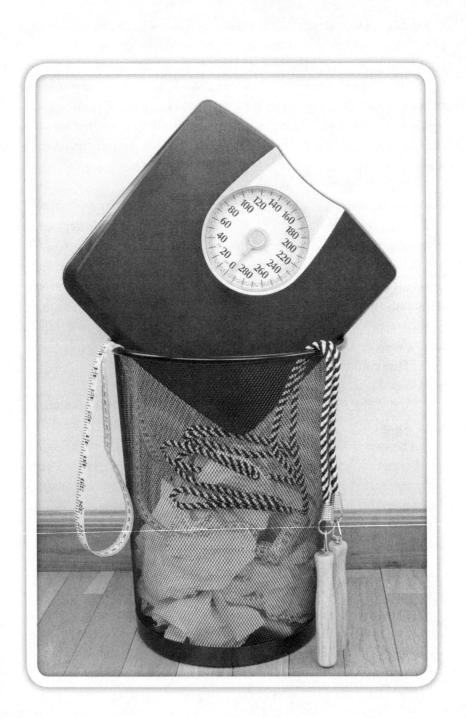

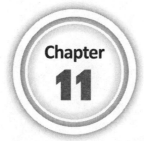

Chapter

11

Curvy & Confident

Proud, Pretty, and Powerful

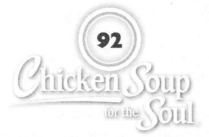

92

Big As Mountain

Always be a first rate version of yourself and not a
second rate version of someone else.
~Judy Garland

I t was my second year of university and I needed a good
summer job to help with the tuition. A dear friend saw my
predicament and invited me to go home with her to Calgary,
where she said jobs were plentiful and paid well. I happily
packed up my few belongings and flew off to Alberta, where my
friend's family greeted us.

They were warm and generous people and treated me as one of
their own from the moment I walked in the door. The next day, I was
on the hunt for a job, full of hope and home-cooked Indian food.

A few days later, while trudging from restaurant to restaurant
with résumés in hand, I was approached by a talent scout from a local
modeling agency.

It had happened before — I am close to six feet tall and due to a
recent struggle with anorexia, was fairly slim at that time. While I had
recovered and since achieved a healthy BMI, I was still occasionally
"spotted" and invited to attend agency screenings. I was skeptical,
suspecting that the agency would be running the same scam that I
had heard three times before — an offer to get me into the industry if I
paid a one-thousand-dollar "training" fee. Waving away my suspicions
and reassuring me with a laugh that everything was above board, the
scout insisted that I should come by.

Proud, Pretty, and Powerful |

With no other jobs in sight, I thought of the money I might be able to make doing local runway shows or commercials. Cautiously, I agreed to the meeting.

That night, over dinner, my new family was not happy. My friend's dad kept saying, in his heavily accented English, "Those beauty ideas are no good! Better you should not go. Don't be sick again!"

Sadly, I agreed with him. But my thoughts were filled with dollar bills and the hope that I could pay for one more year of school.

True to their kind nature, my friend and her dad drove me to the agency the next afternoon and waited outside, supporting my decision while reminding me, "You can leave if you don't like! Remember!"

With my stomach in knots, I took an elevator up to a well-appointed office, complete with expensive works of art and high-end furniture. Intimidated, I waited in silence until I was greeted by a woman who was so thin that she made my heart ache. She introduced herself as an aide to the head of the agency, and asked me to follow her. The beautiful jewelry and silk dress she wore could not hide her jutting collarbones and haggard face. She was my height, but about 30 pounds lighter. Her knees were the thickest part of her legs and her forearms were only as wide as her wrists.

> *"I am not overweight,"* *I suddenly announced, surprising even myself. "This is nonsense."*

I was taken to an inner office where a generously proportioned man sat with an expectant look on his face. He barely greeted me before he placed his hands on his desk and said, "Well, you're a little bit overweight, aren't you?"

It was true. For a model, I was slightly too heavy, and I was certainly curvier than the woman who had escorted me into the office. My struggle against my eating disorder suddenly seemed silly, and perhaps even self-indulgent. Embarrassed, I blushed and said nothing.

What followed was one of the most humiliating thirty minutes I have ever endured. I was measured over my clothes, told that I was "out of shape" and informed that something needed to be done with my nose. At one point the man sat forward, his large belly pressing against the desk, his lip slightly curled as if in disgust.

"I will take you on," he said, as though conceding a point to me, "but there is a condition. I must be the one to control your diet and exercise program. You're just too large."

He then shook his head and launched into a lecture about size and appearance. As the minutes crawled by, I became more and more ashamed of myself, nodding quietly as he ticked off my body flaws on his fingers.

And then his aide walked back in the room, carrying a snack for her boss.

I looked at her, the late afternoon sun washing over her painfully thin face and wasted body, and something in my heart sparked into life.

This woman, I knew, was just as sick as I had been only a year before, and there, accepting his coffee and biscuits without even a nod in her direction, was a man who outweighed the both of us put together. The spark in my heart became a fire.

"I am not overweight," I suddenly announced, surprising even myself. "This is nonsense."

Silence fell over the room. I stood, hoisted my purse to my shoulder and added "And there is absolutely nothing wrong with my nose."

Shaking, I marched out of the office, leaving the man with an astonished expression on his face and a cookie halfway to his mouth.

Down in the car I cried. With humiliated sobs, I recounted the whole fiasco. My friend put her arm around my shoulder as her father listened quietly.

With a hiccup, I added, "And what's worse, I think I was rude."

My friend's father shook his head and looked at me in the rearview mirror.

"No," he said firmly. "No! You should not be ashamed! You should feel big as mountain for putting that man in his place!"

I began to laugh, tears still running down my cheeks. My friend nodded.

"He's right, love," she said, hugging me close. "That was awful, and totally not right for you. Seriously, there are lots of better jobs you can get, okay? And none of them will make you sick again."

Eventually, I did find a job. I waited tables at a little restaurant, and returned to school the following semester—and the one after that too. Paying for school was a struggle, but I found a way through, one waitressing gig at a time. As to my weight—well, deep inside every recovered anorexic there is a nasty little voice that jeers and taunts, that shames and humiliates. Sometimes it sounds like your own voice, sometimes it sounds like someone else, but it's always hurtful and mean. It whispers that food is poison, that weight is weakness, and that curves are ugly.

But since my summer in Calgary so long ago, whenever that hateful murmur echoes through my heart, it is always met by a firm and distinctly accented voice, saying: "Big as mountain! You should feel big as mountain for not letting them win!"

~Alexes Lilly

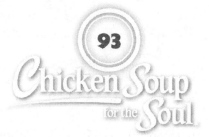

93

Big, Beautiful Heroines

I am always naturally drawn to heroines that have
human flaws because I enjoy people that have
lived their life with courage and make big
successes and big failures.
~Romola Garai

I was eleven years old when I saw my first height/weight chart in a women's magazine, and even though I wasn't a teenager yet, I started judging my body by an adult woman's guidelines. Therein followed twenty-two years of yo-yo dieting, to the point that I was near death. I went on my last diet — the one that almost killed me — when my only child, my son, was three years old. I lost 60 pounds in ten months. And basically every day I had the nervous shakes and a headache. During that time I kept asking, "Why am I doing this to myself?"

Finally, I decided to stop. I realized that my true self lay in my heart and my mind. My body was just the package that I was wrapped in.

From that time forward, I determined that I would, without dieting, eat as healthily each day as I could, without being obsessive about it. I would be as active as I chose to be each day, and with a very active three-year-old that wasn't hard to do.

But most of all, I promised myself that I would start dressing myself to look the best that I could each day. From that point forward, I never left my house without my clothes, hair and make-up done the way I liked them.

This wasn't hard for me because I'd always loved to play "dress up." But as I'd gained more and more weight after the birth of my son, I'd fallen into a pattern of wearing clothes that didn't make me feel confident. So, even though we didn't have much free cash at the time, I went shopping and bought a few new items of clothing that were designed for my larger body.

Up until this moment in my life, I had no idea what my adult body would look like if I didn't diet. So I determined to love the body that developed, whatever size it was. I also determined that I would hold my head up, shoulders back, and show the world that I loved who I was.

> *"You can love me just like I am, or you can stay away from me."*

And a remarkable thing happened. Almost every time I went out in public, a stranger would give me a compliment. I began to realize that my *looks* hadn't changed; it was my *opinion* of myself that had changed. And as I learned to love, respect, and enjoy my body, my confidence grew and grew and grew.

I can't explain the pure joy that began to surge through me as this newfound "self" was developing. There was such a freedom! I no longer cared if someone secretly judged me, because I was larger than they thought I should be.

I developed an entirely new attitude. I became a size-acceptance activist. Very seldom did anyone say anything about my weight, but when they did, I carefully explained to them that this was my weight and not their concern.

For example, I was at a church function and an older woman kept telling me how beautiful I was. She went on and on, until I was actually getting a little tired of it. Then she said, "If you would only lose 70 pounds, you'd be a knockout!" I remember leaning over to her and whispering for her ears only, "You can love me just like I am, or you can stay away from me."

I also started taking on anyone who dared to say something negative about someone else's larger body. I let nothing pass. Friends, family, strangers, ministers, letters to magazine editors, letters to the editor of my local newspaper… nobody was safe from me and my one-person campaign to educate the world about weight issues.

Furthermore, I stopped allowing anyone to stand in my presence and say negative things about themselves.

Soon, I began to see that there were very few positive role models for larger-sized women in the movies, magazines, novels or anywhere. Basically, anytime a larger woman was mentioned in these outlets it was in a negative way.

So, having always loved to write, and having always planned to write a novel at some point, I decided to write a novel with what I called a Big Beautiful Heroine. But I soon realized that the major publishers were afraid to take a chance on this type of novel, because these books might not bring in the kind of money that they wanted.

So I self-published my first four books, then found a small publisher that wanted my books. At the present time, including the book I just sent to the publisher, I will have thirteen fiction and non-fiction books published on learning to love the body that you have.

My main theme is to encourage people of all sizes to love the body that they have and stop trying to be or look like someone that they're not genetically programmed to be.

The one phrase that I use constantly is, "You are a one-of-a-kind work of art. There never has been, and there never will be another you. So love the unique being that you are."

~Pat Ballard

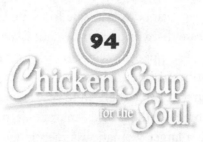

94

Tall Boots

*Remember always that you not only have the right to
be an individual, you have an obligation to be one.*
~Eleanor Roosevelt

I may not be the image in most magazines
Yet and still, I am queen
Never needed designer jeans
I stand tall with self-esteem
I won't let society bring me down
I won't shed tears or be your clown
I am she with radio voice
The local viewers' choice
Striving for a Rolls-Royce
These curves wrecked nerves
Back in the day it was just my way
My smile, my style, my lips and these hips
I am fully equipped like a limousine
Filled with high octane gasoline
As I stated I am queen
My heart is kind, my arms are wide
My emotions I dare not hide
Please don't tell me my face is pretty again
I am pleased with my beauty within
I am completely adorable
Extremely witty, like those ladies

From *Sex in the City*
I am a food for the soul
Not a happy little meal
With mass appeal, (just keeping it real)
I am vintage, not old
Take a closer look
When it comes to confidence
I wrote the book with my own chapter
It's entitled, Love & Laughter
That's what I'm after
My boots are tall, my dreams are bigger
When I step to the mic, I truly deliver
Never apologize for your size
Disregard those staring eyes
Hold your head high when you enter a room
Be proud with or without a groom
Keep mind, body and spirit in tune
Sip lemon water on a hot afternoon
Admire the stars, the sun and moon
Stand in your truth and be not afraid
Know that your path has been paved
You are like most of us
P.L.U.S.
Pretty, Loving, Unique and Sweet
There are no lost lyrics on my song
I am simply here to re-write the wrongs
I dress nicely — red hair, freckles and all
I love my curves and my boots are tall

~Jimmie Ware

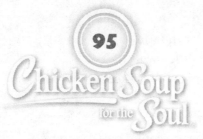

95

The Milkshake Diet

*Too many people overvalue what they are not and
undervalue what they are.*
~Malcolm S. Forbes

I wasn't overweight as a teenager. In fact, the other kids would call me "skinny," "bony," and "toothpick." They made fun of me for having no figure at all. When I was the fragile age of fourteen and still undeveloped, a boy stood up in class and demonstrated my flat as a board, shapeless figure to all the kids in my class. Everyone roared with laughter. I felt like sinking through the floor.

My mother became so concerned about my abnormal, underweight physique that she brought me to the doctor, who took a look at me and prescribed daily milkshakes. I followed his instructions but still didn't gain much weight. How could I since I never ate a compete meal? I picked at the chicken or pasta or vegetables on my plate, because I had no real interest in healthy, nourishing food. I lived on a diet of doctor-ordered milkshakes, soda, chocolate cookies, and the occasional can of soup thrown in for nutrition.

That all changed when I met my husband. In our second year of marriage we lived with his family, who had healthy appetites. My sister-in-law was an amazing cook and prepared fabulous meals. I soon learned to appreciate the taste of real food. I ate entire juicy chuck steaks, eggs with buttered toast, seasoned roasted chicken, fluffy rice, and baked potatoes slathered in sour cream and butter. We devoured rich desserts every night — apple pies, frosted cakes, cookies, cannolis, and a freezer loaded with every flavor of ice cream. Second helpings were encouraged. There were no scales at their house, and I started to put on weight. Soon, I looked in the mirror and didn't recognize my reflection.

My friends told me about their diets. My mom was upset with me and told me I needed to watch my weight. My husband teased me about my expanding body. I didn't feel pretty. But that was no surprise; I never felt pretty when I was skinny, either.

I gave birth to four beautiful children, and with each child I put on more weight. I'd bake them treats, and take some for myself. I made pies from scratch. When they didn't finish their meals, I finished for them. After all, I couldn't let good food go to waste.

My marriage ended in divorce and I began eating from the stress of being a single parent. Whenever I'd get angry or upset, I'd reach for the potato chips and eat half a bag before I realized what I was doing.

That is, until one day, I had heart palpitations and my cardiologist told me I was obese. I was shocked. He warned me that if I didn't start developing healthier food and exercise habits, I would develop serious health issues.

I began dieting in earnest and working out on the treadmill three times a week. I lost 38 pounds and I looked amazing… for a year. But I still didn't feel pretty.

When my mother became seriously ill, food became my best friend again. Within a year, I'd gained all the weight back.

I felt horrible. I was disappointed in myself and I stopped caring about my appearance. I wore old, dark clothes and it was an effort every single day to get up and dressed.

Then one evening, I had a defining moment.

I was out with some friends and saw a curvy, confident woman dancing with her husband, laughing with him on the dance floor. They were clearly in love, and I discovered they had been happily married for years. She was wearing gorgeous, bright clothes, while I sat in the corner shrinking out of sight in my black outfit, a desperate attempt to hide my extra pounds.

After that, something really cool happened. I started seeing them everywhere, these gorgeous, curvy, beautiful women who danced at parties and worked out at gyms and ate healthy diets, indulging in reasonable portions of scrumptious desserts. And they had partners who loved them unconditionally — just as they were.

> *I started seeing them everywhere, these gorgeous, curvy, beautiful women who danced at parties and worked out at gyms and ate healthy diets.*

Wait. Weren't we supposed to be thin? But these women were living amazing lives full of love and all of them were carrying extra pounds. They had the lives that I craved.

As women, we are assaulted daily by magazines spewing out diet plans and magic weight loss pills, claiming they will transform our lives. We gaze at airbrushed models who make us feel inferior. It's time to ignore these negative messages, and love ourselves the way we were made.

One day, I looked at myself in the mirror, with all my curves and all the extra pounds, and I felt love for myself — for the first time. I looked straight into my own eyes. "You're beautiful," I said, "Exactly the way you are."

And when I began to love my body, I began to love myself.

~L.A. Strucke

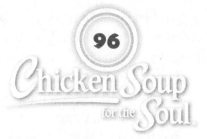

The Look

Taking joy in living is a woman's best cosmetic.
~Rosalind Russell

"Good evening," the baritone voice behind me boomed. I set the eggs down on the conveyor belt and slowly turned to identify the source of the voice. It was the handsome gentleman I had noticed earlier while I raced through the store. He stood about 6'3" and wore a Cleveland Cavaliers shirt, required attire in my city following the team's first NBA finals win.

"Hello, how are you?" I said with a grin. He smiled back and gave me "the look."

My girlfriends are skinny and drop-dead gorgeous, so guys always gave them "the look" when we were out. It was the special way a man looked deeply into a woman's eyes and grinned. Usually it was my friends getting "the look," but today it was me. Size 18 me.

Workout clothes. Hair in a ponytail. No make-up. Possible stench coming from my underarms after a four-mile power walk.

Five years ago my first reaction would have been to curse myself for stopping by the store while looking so shabby. But five years ago my workout clothes would have consisted of super-sized jogging pants from the men's department and an old family reunion T-shirt.

Today, I had on a bright orange V-neck — fitted enough that it didn't look like the tents I used to wear, loose enough that my rolls of fat weren't waving at passersby. The black workout capris stopped mid-calf, highlighting my best feature if I do say so myself. My sisterlocks were pulled into a ponytail that cascaded down my back. I had grown more comfortable with leaving the house without make-up since my daily four-mile walks in the sunshine had given my caramel skin a deep mocha glow. Even after working out, I looked cute!

"I'm doing well. It's a beautiful day out, isn't it?" he asked.

"Yes, not too hot. It was a great day for a walk." Yep, he was definitely giving me "the look." I turned back to unloading my cart so he wouldn't see me blush. I was so proud of myself for even responding. I used to dismiss any attention I received from men because I assumed there was no way a man could be attracted to a plus-size woman like me.

My journey to self-confidence had begun a few years earlier.

At the encouragement of my friend, Maria, I had joined an online dating site, indicating on my profile that I was plus-sized and posting a full-body photo. I was convinced no one would respond. My past experience with boys and men taught me that they were not attracted to large women, and specifically not me. I was convinced that as long as I was overweight, I was perpetually unattractive.

But I did get some responses, and when it came time to meet one of my potential suitors for a date, Maria took me shopping for an outfit. One by one, I rejected every item of clothing she suggested, and she finally said what she must have been thinking for years: "You dress like an old church lady, and you are only in your thirties!"

She was right about how I dressed, and I knew it. I hesitantly agreed to her choice — a bright blue sweater and multi-colored leggings.

When I walked into the coffee shop to meet my date for the first time, he stood as I approached and you guessed it — he gave me "the look." He continued to gaze at me intently throughout the evening, and on every date we had after that. Each time I saw him he'd greet me with that pleased look on his face and compliment me.

We didn't end up being a match, but at thirty-seven I was happy to have had my first adult dating experience with a good guy who liked size 18 me enough to give me the you-know-what.

Each man since then who has given me "the look" or has taken the time to tell me that I was beautiful has helped me reconstruct a counter narrative to the one I had developed over the years about my so-called non-attractiveness. I always knew that God said I was fearfully and wonderfully made, and now I understand that others see that beauty as well.

> *Now, when a man gives me "the look"—I believe it.*

And now when the voice of doubt tries to tell me that all men are disgusted by my appearance, I argue back and say, "I have evidence to the contrary!"

Now, I can rock a bright orange top when I work out. Now, when a man gives me "the look" — I believe it.

I paid the cashier and loaded the bags in my cart.

On my way out I turned back to the tall Cavaliers fan, who smiled and said, "You have a good evening now."

I would.

~J. Renee

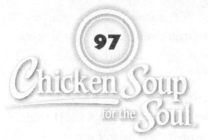

97

Big Girl, Big World

To be yourself in a world that is constantly trying to make you something else is the greatest accomplishment.

~Ralph Waldo Emerson

I was sitting at my desk in a great mood when a co-worker casually walked by my cubby. "Hey, I never noticed before," he said, "but you're pretty cute... for a big girl."

It was a backhanded compliment I'd heard before, and I'm sure he thought he was flattering me. But adding anything after "cute" was unnecessary and an insult and just plain rude. "Cute" and "big" are not mutually exclusive, and attractiveness isn't determined by size.

I can't remember my response, but I'm sure it was something like: "I'm cute... *period.*"

I was tormented in my youth for not fitting into "normal" sized clothes. I had to have my choir dresses special ordered because they were plus-sized, and my teacher had to alter the dance moves in a routine one time because my partner could not lift me up at the end of the number.

At home, my stepfather teased that he would have to pay someone to escort me to senior prom. (He didn't, but fearing that reality for four years did a lot of emotional damage.)

As a "minority" you find ways to cope. I made sure to perform — I was always "on", singing and dancing and making people laugh. It masked the hurt of my heaviness.

It wasn't until college that I was seen as a person, not defined by weight or color, but for my personality. College was a different world. I was catcalled, whistled at, and guys approached me with genuine interest. At first, I didn't know how to process it. I thought I was the dare they lost or a prank that would later blow up in my face, but the other shoe never dropped.

"You're pretty cute... for a big girl."

My college experiences helped me grow and taught me the value of self-worth and love. Now size, just like age, is nothing but a number. I know I look good and my fiancé threatens to leave me if I lose too much weight. He says I "barely made the (weight) requirement."

I make sure I eat right and I'm working on exercising more. I feel good, I look good and I am good. And I will continue to educate the uninformed that just because I am big, it doesn't make everything else about me small.

To the universe at large, I am only a grain of sand, so, in fact, my bigness is insignificant. But I am a force to be reckoned with.

And I'm cute. Period.

~Shantell Antoinette

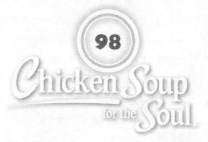

98

I Am Delicious!

Grandmother-grandchild relationships are simple.
Grandmas are short on criticism and long on love.
~Author Unknown

"Eat, eat, eat," my little Hungarian grandmother ordered as she pushed a second walnut stuffed kiffle in front of me while adding more butter into the dough she was blending at her kitchen table.

"This will be a special batch for you to take home," she said with a smile that filled her face. Her chant, combined with an old-country accent, continued, "Eat, you are too thin!" This became an almost religious mantra in my grandmother's household. "Eat, eat, eat," developed an insatiable rhythm of its own as you stuffed oversized portions of her delicacies into your mouth.

"Grandma," I argued, "I am not too thin. All the girls in school call me fat and make fun of me." Fourth grade was a wicked year for me. I was too young to flirt with boys and too old to play with dolls, and I lived in this elementary-school limbo in which I was intimidated by classmates who, in my eyes, looked perfect!

"Did you know that Mom has to go to a special store to buy my uniform? They only sell clothes for 'huskies.' Do you know what size that is? Huskies are for fat girls," I screamed.

Without interrupting her task of rolling the kiffle dough, she said calmly, "Husky, isn't that a cute dog that people love to cuddle?"

"Okay, so there are two meanings," I said, "but the other meaning is fat, you know, big, large, heavy, fat!" I yelled so loud the next-door neighbor stopped watering his garden and ran inside.

"Fat?" she questioned. "What is fat? There is only one meaning for fat in Hungarian, and that is something that makes food delicious," she said, as she stirred the special walnut mixture that would plump up her crescent-shaped kiffles. Then, she ordered me to follow her. While wiping her hands on her handmade apron, she marched me to her bedroom and stood me in front of her beautiful, ornate mirror. Taking her brush from her bureau, she brushed my hair away from my face.

> *Real beauty comes from the heart. I see yours and it's beautiful.*

"Look deep in the mirror," she said. "Who do you see?" Of course, being focused only on myself, I never noticed her little, round body next to mine.

It took a while for me to answer. "I see an ugly girl, Grandma," I sighed, "a very fat, ugly girl." And then I cried.

She pulled me close to her soft, comfortable body. "No, no, no," she said, as my tears fell onto her apron. She wiped them gently away with her wrinkled, embroidered hanky, and continued. "Look deeper. I see two beautiful ladies, a young one and an old one. The young one is just starting to understand what real beauty is all about, and the old one already knows because she has lived long enough. Real beauty comes from the heart. I see yours and it's beautiful. One day, you will understand."

With that reflection, she returned to her kitchen table and invited me to eat yet another walnut stuffed kiffle while firmly saying, "When those girls in school call you fat, just tell them you are delicious!"

Despite all the anxious conversations I had with my grandmother about being overweight, I never saw *her* that way. Her soft curves cushioned babies, comforted tears, and hugged multitudes of family and friends who needed to know they were loved.

My grandmother died many years ago. I am trying to age gracefully, accepting the added wrinkles and pounds that are captured in the mirror that once was hers. Some days, when I stand in front of it, I

Proud, Pretty, and Powerful |

still see my little, round grandmother standing next to me. I remember her treasured, encouraging words: "You are not fat, you are delicious!"

A confident, beautiful smile brightens my face because I finally understand her meaning of those heartfelt words, and yes, I am delicious!

~Lainie Belcastro

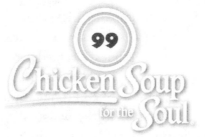

99

It Took Time to Love My Hourglass Figure

*Our self-respect tracks our choices. Every time we act
in harmony with our authentic self and our heart,
we earn our respect. It is that simple.
Every choice matters.*
~Dan Coppersmith

I was seven years old the first time someone called me "fat." A family member told me that I couldn't have any dessert and when I asked why, I was told, "You're already fat. You don't need any more food." Little did I know at that time, I had many more years of emotional abuse to come.

At nine years old, a lot of the boys and girls in my grade and the grades above me began to tease me for being "fat." They wouldn't let me play with them at recess and some of them even pretended to be my friend so that they could tell the others my secrets. The words and actions of my school peers got worse over time.

I turned to food to comfort myself. I went from chubby to overweight from fourth to fifth grade. And that was when I decided to start dieting. I stopped eating breakfast, and when no one noticed, I started skipping lunch too. I ate one small meal a day, usually two granola bars, until I was twelve years old, but I didn't lose weight. At thirteen years old, I stopped eating altogether, and if I did eat, I would run to the bathroom to try to "un-do" what I just did.

At fourteen years old I was eating two hundred calories a day and obsessing over models in magazines. I wanted to be skin and bones like them. I thought more people would like me. Despite starving myself, I couldn't get below a size 10, which I thought was unacceptable.

The high school years were the worst. With the explosion of instant messenger and texting, I became a target of cyber bullying. People sent mean messages to me about how I should kill myself, stop eating, etc. all because I was different than them. I tried so hard to fit in during high school that I strayed far away from who I actually was. I didn't even recognize myself anymore. And to protect myself, I started being mean to other people. The meaner I was to people, the less they would be mean to me, I thought. It made it worse because I felt so horrible about being cruel to people.

> *I have learned to love the body that I was genetically destined to have.*

The years of eating so little finally caught up to me, too. I began to suffer some ugly side effects of malnutrition. I was always tired, my nails were brittle, and my hair began to fall out. That was my wake-up call. I finally reached out to get help.

My therapist worked extremely hard with me until one day I woke up and accepted the fact that I will always have an hourglass figure and there's nothing wrong with that. It took many sessions of resistance, crying, and doubt, but, once I realized that my hourglass figure is something to love, it was like seeing a rainbow after a terrible storm.

Asking for help was one of the greatest things that I did for myself. Once I stopped counting calories, visiting the bathroom, and putting myself down, I stopped hating myself. For the first time in years, I was able to eat in public, I was able to be at the beach or pool in a bathing suit without thinking that everyone was staring, and I was able to love myself again.

The journey to loving my curves was a bumpy road, but I have learned to love the body that I was genetically destined to have. I still have my moments of self-consciousness, but I have a wonderful support system to remind me that the extra weight that I carry is nothing compared to the love I can give and receive from the world.

~Nicole F. Anderson

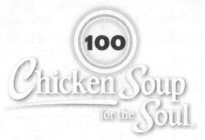

100

The Beauty Within

Real beauty is to be true to oneself. That's
what makes me feel good.
~Laetitia Casta

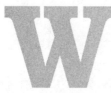hen I was growing up, there was always something good cooking or baking in the kitchen: Sunday sauce and meatballs, roast beef with mashed potatoes and peas, lasagna, pumpkin pie and brownies for dessert.

My parents, who've been lovingly married for forty-five years, contributed to my strong sense of wellbeing, emotional health and body image. My father always told my mother how beautiful she was no matter what size she was and my siblings and I were always told how wonderful we were. My parents were caring and respectful of each other and of us; they were great role models for how to treat ourselves and others.

That's why it was hard for me to understand how overwhelming my body issues became after giving birth to my son when I was eighteen. Pre-baby, I was 5'11", size 10 and 145 pounds. I assumed I would be thin forever. I wasn't prepared for the whopping 77 pounds I gained in those nine months.

It took me twenty-four years to accept that it wasn't just a baby that changed my body — it was also being a working, single mother, with all the accompanying emotions: guilt, fear, loneliness, and exhaustion. I dealt with my emotions by eating. An extra serving of fried chicken always worked, right?

As time went on, society seemed more judgmental about women and their bodies. And I hadn't changed my childhood eating habits. I was still treating myself to cereal, sodas, ice cream, baked potatoes, pizza, pumpkin pie and lasagna — all the foods I thought were "fun" and symbolized good times, holidays, and weekends. I worked long days as a florist and that meant unscheduled eating and quick, feel-good, cheap meals most nights.

The stress of being a single mom and running a small business affected me deeply. I began to feel as though I didn't deserve to be happy or loved. But food never let me down or made me sad.

My father always told my mother how beautiful she was no matter what size she was.

After my son left for college, I felt lost. It got worse when he subsequently joined the United States Marine Corps.

But it wasn't until one very long, emotionally draining romantic relationship ended badly that I took control of my life. The end of the romance made me realize that I had to stop letting other people decide if I was beautiful. My weight did not define my beauty inside or out. And most importantly, I realized that I deserved more for myself. I was going to put myself first. I finally accepted that I was the only one responsible for my happiness.

I started riding my bike down to the beach and to and from work. The exercise helped me get through those long days at work and helped me with all the emotions of missing my son. I started to eat salads and more vegetables and fish. I cut out sodas, snacks, and pastas. I bought books on detoxing and sugar. If my son could endure becoming a Marine, I thought, then I could work out and make healthy choices and go to his boot camp graduation 20 pounds lighter.

I wanted to make him proud of me.

I joined a cross-fit gym and loved it. It was hard, but they were kind and motivating. I learned how one's body reacts to weightlifting and a healthy diet. I was focused. I felt amazing. And after only a few weeks, I was down 8 pounds!

Proud, Pretty, and Powerful | 339

But it wasn't really about the weight, it was about a shift in my core. I felt stronger, inside and out. I was making better choices with the food I put in my body and seeing the results in glowing skin, better sleep, and more energy.

It's now four years later, and I'm happy to report that I am in love — with myself, with my life, and with the most genuine, wonderful, loving and supportive man I have ever met. We ride bikes together, we cook, and we laugh. Being happy has done wonders for my figure. And, like my father did for my mother, he makes me feel beautiful every day, no matter what size I am.

My son, who is an inspiration to me, returned home after serving four years in the military. At home, we don't eat processed foods and I have an organic vegetable garden.

Once in a while, I indulge in some good old-fashioned fried chicken. But mostly, I surround myself with healthy food, good people, work I'm proud of, and lots and lots of beautiful flowers.

I don't feel plus size; I feel *my* size.

~Jenny Wildflower

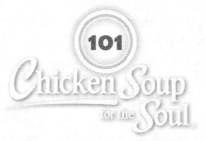

Go Ahead, Look at Me

A successful person is one who can lay a firm
foundation with the bricks that others
throw at him or her.
~David Brinkley

As we were putting the final touches on *Chicken Soup for the Soul: Curvy & Confident*, Amy, Emme, and I — three relatively confident blondes of varied curviness — met for well-deserved cocktails at a swanky hotel on Central Park South. It was late afternoon on a Friday and we were relaxing together after many weeks of reading and re-reading the stories for this book.

"I want to meet our contributors and hug them," I said, as we toasted. "They are so brave and vulnerable to tell such personal stories." Some of the anecdotes about body shaming had touched me so much, I cried while reading them.

Emme had been all over the news the week before talking about that very issue. Republican presidential candidate Donald Trump had complained about the weight gained by Miss Universe Alicia Machado during her reign, and a lot of people were offended and outraged.

"How can he think this is okay?" Emme asked. "This is completely unacceptable behavior."

We were all silent for a moment, as Amy and Emme looked at me.

"Natasha," Amy said quietly, "when are you going to write about your Trump experience?"

Ah yes. *That*. It was a question Amy had been asking for months, ever since I'd stayed at her house in the spring while coaching her through writing her first solo book, *Simply Happy*. We'd seen Trump on TV pounding the election trail and I had told her what The Donald had done a decade earlier. Emme had known the story ever since it happened in 2005.

Back then, I'd gone to the Trumps' Mar-a-Lago estate in Palm Beach to interview them for a *People* magazine feature and there, Trump had cornered me alone in a room and forcibly kissed, then propositioned, me while his pregnant wife was upstairs.

"Maybe I should, but I'm afraid to," I said. "Look what he does to women."

As if on cue, one of our cell phones buzzed with breaking news: A tape had surfaced in which candidate Trump was heard speaking crudely about women and their body parts, describing doing exactly the same kind of thing he had done to me.

"It's time, Natasha," both Amy and Emme urged.

Except for a circle of trusted friends, family, and colleagues whom I told at the time, I'd kept mostly quiet about the incident. I had many good reasons to do so. And there was something else lingering at the back of my mind: Trump was known for viciously attacking women's looks when he didn't like them or when he wanted to intimidate them — the term "fat pig" rings in my ears as one term he's fond of using. I was worried he'd do the same to me and it would be a blow to my hard-earned positive body image.

That had been my history: When one family member told me I had the shoulders of a linebacker, I started slouching. When another said my legs were too strong, I stopped wearing skirts. Color me overly sensitive, but I think many of the writers in this book can relate. We have more than a few stories in these pages about harmful, hurtful words uttered by parents, siblings, friends, classmates, and strangers that have caused a lot of pain.

I'd already spent years feeling ashamed and degraded by his actions and words and I didn't want to subject myself to any more humiliation, especially in front of the entire world.

Skip ahead one week, and that's exactly what happened.

Two days after our girls' night out, Trump appeared on the second debate and denied ever kissing a woman without her consent. This statement pushed the issue to its tipping point for me and several other women who decided to come forward. *People* approached me to tell my story, and I said yes. Three days later, it went online on their website.

A lot of thought — more than a decade's worth — and many conversations with editors, my family and friends went into the decision. And also, so did my experience working on this book. I'd been inspired by the hundreds of personal anecdotes I'd read about women empowering themselves and not allowing other people's limited, skewed concepts of beauty interfere with how they thought about themselves. I knew Trump would probably attack my appearance no matter what I looked like, but I took the risk anyway and came forward. If our *Curvy & Confident* writers could be brave and bare their souls, so could I.

> *Even when you are trying to be a brave woman and stand up for yourself, it stings to be attacked for your appearance.*

A day and a half after the story posted, Trump implied to supporters at a rally in Florida that I *wasn't attractive enough* to sexually assault. Now there's an insult I hadn't heard before. Or was it a compliment?

"Take a look at her! You tell me what you think!" he yelled to the crowd. "*I don't think so!*" The next day he called me a liar and told everyone, "*Check out her Facebook page. You'll understand.*"

Gulp. This sort of thing can bruise a girl's ego.

There was no way I was going to do any TV interviews about this story. *People* and Chicken Soup for the Soul and other friends were fielding requests for me from *CNN, Today, Anderson Cooper, Good Morning America* and more.

But besides the fact that I'd said my piece and didn't want to talk about it anymore (I wasn't, to quote Trump's words during the final presidential debate, seeking my "ten minutes of fame"), I didn't want to put myself out there on camera and invite even more scorn and insults from him. Some articles suggested Trump attacked his accusers' looks to discourage other women from coming forward. I'm sure his words did have that effect. Even when you are trying to be brave and stand up for yourself, it stings to be attacked for your appearance.

I stayed silent for a week after the story went online, hidden away in a hotel in New Jersey finishing my work on this book and working on my next book, too. My friends protected me, and my privacy. Meanwhile, I took comfort in the hundreds of supportive e-mails and online comments from women whose confidence had been shaken by similar experiences.

But Trump had challenged my credibility, so *People* decided to publish a follow-up story—interviews from close friends and colleagues I'd told the story to back in 2005. It was important for me and for all the other women out there that my story be corroborated.

This meant I had to come out of hiding and pose for at least one photo. The pictures of me used in news stories and blogs all over the Internet had been grabs from my Facebook page before I shut it down—old selfies and pics taken by friends (one was taken by Emme the day I accompanied her to the hospital for chemo)—and the magazine needed something up-to-date. I felt self-conscious about it, but I agreed.

I met the photographer in a loft in Chelsea and we got to work. Her assistant put on Frank Sinatra ballads, the make-up artist curled my lashes, and I posed. I tried not to think about the reality that millions of people would be scrutinizing this photo, including you-know-who. No pressure! I tried to look good, I tried to look confident, and I held my head up high. As I did this, something surprisingly wonderful happened.

I was a photojournalist in the early days of my career, and I can tell you that the camera doesn't lie. What you see through the lens is what you get; it is truth.

The *People* photographer saw it too.

"Confidence!" she yelled out. "Yes!"

I smiled. She was right. It felt good to overcome my fear and do the right thing. It felt good to reclaim my power from him. It didn't matter what nasty things he said about me. I would no longer let the words, opinions, or actions of one person, any person, hurt me. I was serene, confident, and empowered.

So go ahead, look at me.

~Natasha Stoynoff

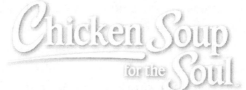

Afterword

I was first introduced to Emme by our mutual friend, Natasha Stoynoff. We had been talking about making this book since late 2015 and it was time to meet in person. So on the last day of January 2016, a Sunday, my husband drove me down to the diner across from the YMCA in our town, where I was to meet the famous Emme.

Ironically, I was having the worst flare-up of my bad back in years, so I was barely able to get in and out of the car, which was why Bill had to drive me. I crept up the diner's front steps, hunched over and pulling myself up by gripping the railing. And there was Emme waiting for me in a booth, sitting tall and strong in her workout clothes, with her wet, blond hair pulled straight back from her face that was flushed from swimming laps at the Y. Boy did I feel weak and small and seriously *un*athletic next to her.

Emme and I talked about one of her key messages — that you should *love* your body, *nurture* your body, and *use* your body. She talked about how you need to integrate your mind and your body, and view yourself as one whole being, not a person who has a brain and then has this *appendage* — a body.

When we came up with this book idea, we had no idea how topical it would turn out to be. Before we knew it, in early 2016, Mattel was introducing Curvy Barbie, *Sports Illustrated* was featuring plus-size and "real" women in its swimsuit issue, and Lane Bryant was covering the sides of buses with plus-size models wearing fun, colorful clothing for larger women — no more shapeless, black tunics.

It seemed to Emme, Natasha, and I that we were really onto

something. Every time we turned around we heard a global conversation about body image, realistic portrayal of women, healthy eating, and a new more constructive view of natural beauty. We were thrilled with the thousands of stories that were submitted for this collection and we knew they would be an important part of this movement to clearer thinking.

But we returned to negative talk in a HUGE way during the presidential campaign in the fall, with Donald Trump repeatedly denigrating women for their appearance. We learned that the still gorgeous Alicia Machado was denounced by him for having gained weight after she won the Miss Universe pageant at age nineteen — or, dare I say, for having returned to a healthier, more realistic weight. And we watched him insult his opponent for how she *looked* from behind, and also insult the appearance of women who came forward with accounts of their treatment at his hands in the past.

We had no idea when we started making this book that our own co-author, Natasha Stoynoff, would end up center stage while we were trying to finish the manuscript. She didn't want to go public — one reason among many was because it would subject her to insults about her appearance, which she knew would be forthcoming — but she reluctantly did so because it was the right thing to do. Emme and I were among those who urged her to end her eleven-year silence. It meant that we would lose a few weeks of editing time, and this book would not make its deadline to the printer, but it was important.

So now, here we are, sending this book to the printer very late, but knowing that our book is even more relevant than we had imagined. This conversation is important, and we are proud to be part of what I like to call The Curvy & Confident Movement.

~Amy Newmark
Editor-in-Chief and Publisher, Chicken Soup for the Soul
October 31, 2016

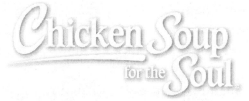

Meet Our Contributors

Tamara Albanna received her bachelor's degree in English Language and Literature, and her master's degree in International Relations. She is the author of *My Name is Inanna*, and also has an upcoming book of poetry. Tamara currently resides in Vienna, Austria with her family.

Andrea Amador is "The Juicy Woman." She's a curvy and confident Professional Empowerment Coach who leads women to step into their power so they can feel worthy and wonderful and sexy and sassy at every size. Andrea is the proud author of the book, *Lovin' the Skin You're In*. Learn more at thejuicywoman.com.

Nicole F. Anderson was born and raised in Chicago, IL. She's currently a college student pursing a degree in journalism and creative writing and is the Editor-in-Chief for her college's newspaper and literary arts magazine.

Darbie Andrews is a single mother of two sons, a bilingual high school teacher, and a teen counselor. She's appeared in various media for her teaching and writing, her work with at-risk teens, and her various charity efforts. She has a B.A. and M.A. degree from University of California, Santa Barbara and California State University, San Bernardino.

Mary Anglin-Coulter received her Bachelor of Arts degree from Bellarmine University. In early 2016, she quit her job to start a freelance writing and graphic design business and is working on her first book. This is her fourth contribution to the *Chicken Soup for the Soul* series. Mary is married with three children. E-mail her at mary@anglincoulter.com.

Shantell Antoinette is a recent transplant to Rock Hill, SC by way of Cleveland, OH. Shantell is a spoken word artist, published author, singer/songwriter and performing artist. She and her husband, Leonard Johnson, share a love for poetry and music, combining this love to form the poetry duo, Eight Sideways.

Violetta Armour is a former English teacher and bookstore owner. She published her debut novel *I'll Always Be with You* in 2015, which has become a book club favorite. She would love to Skype with your book group. Contact her through her blog at serendipity-reflections. blogspot.com.

Elizabeth Atwater lives on a horse ranch with her husband Joe in a small town in North Carolina. She enjoys tending to her rose garden, reading when she can find a quiet, uninterrupted part of her busy schedule to do so, and writing, of course.

Pat Ballard became a "health at any size" activist after she stopped twenty-two years of dieting. Pat has written and published thirteen books encouraging others to love the body they were born with. Her story and books can be found at patballard.com.

Lainie Belcastro has many titles in the arts, but her most treasured title is mom to her daughter Nika. They are the creators of Mrs. Terra Cotta Pots & Twig, trademarked storytellers, who plant dreams for children. Lainie, a published writer in many genres, is thrilled to share her stories in the *Chicken Soup for the Soul* series!

Melissa Berry is a fashion, beauty and lifestyle publicist and founder of CancerFashionista.com, a valuable fashion and beauty resource for those undergoing breast cancer treatment and beyond. Melissa lives in New Jersey with her two daughters. E-mail her at Melissa@cancerfashionista.com.

Kristina Bigby received her bachelor's degree from the University of Virginia, and her Master's of Journalism degree from the University of Maryland. Kristina, a leading body positive advocate, coined the phrase #ForTheLoveOfCurves. She explores confidence and positive self-esteem on CurvyGirlChronicles.net. She thanks God for her family.

A plus fashion pioneer, **Alexandra Boos** has propelled forward in the industry by working as a model, on-air spokesperson, fashion, fit and brand consultant, fashion show and photo shoot producer as well as Marketing and Creative Director of the top plus fashion magazine. She now is the Curves Director at TRUE Model Management in New York City. In 2016, Alexandra was honored as a LEGEND by FFFWeek.

Joyelle Brandt is a radical self-love warrior. As an artist, author and speaker, she works to help women heal their relationships with their bodies and recover from abuse trauma. She is the author/illustrator of *Princess Monsters from A to Z*, and co-editor of the *Trigger Points* anthology.

Karla Brown attended St. Joseph's University years ago! Married, and living in Pennsylvania, she loves her family, gardening, and adopting cats. Her first novel, *Miss Darling*, will soon be published by Soul Mate Publishing.

Michelle Bruce received her degree and began working as a nurse in 1990. She and her husband Jeremy have four children and enjoy watching their sports and cheerleading. Michelle loves travel, swimming, and flower gardening. Michelle spends her days writing and is currently working on a new book.

Ray Budd taught music for thirty-three years in public school, and then spent seventeen years as a computer programmer at Carnegie

Mellon University. He has been a professional jazz musician all his life and lives with his wife Bernice in Pittsburgh, PA. He also has a story published in the magazine *Good Old Days*.

Jill Burns lives in the mountains of West Virginia with her wonderful family. She's a retired piano teacher and performer. She enjoys writing, music, gardening, nature, and spending time with her grandchildren.

Emily Canning-Dean is a graduate of The University of Akron and works as a reporter for a weekly suburban newspaper. She lives in Ohio with her husband Eric and their cat Mr. Muffins. Emily loves swimming, hanging out with friends and family, and playing cards.

Nicole Caratas is a junior at Saint Mary's College in Notre Dame, IN. She is studying English Writing and Humanistic Studies and serves as the Saint Mary's editor for *The Observer* and the contributing editor for the Saint Mary's *Odyssey*. She enjoys reading, writing, history, good music, puppies, and donuts.

Candace Carteen has been writing since the age of eight. She's a widowed mom with a sixteen-year-old son who's in the entertainment business. He writes for *The Huffington Post*. As he moves on toward college, her writing world becomes bigger to fill in that loss. E-mail her at ccarteeen@gmail.com.

Cindi Carver-Futch specializes in creative nonfiction and short story writing, but is also a technical writer, creative writing mentor, and performer. She has degrees in English and nonprofit management, and when not traveling she lives in Charleston, SC with her husband, daughter, two dogs and an occasional foreign exchange student.

Kathrine Conroy struggled with body image for most of her life before finding yoga. Through yoga, she learned to love herself and her body and learned how strong she can be — mentally and physically.

Priscilla Dann-Courtney is a writer and clinical psychologist living in Boulder, CO. Her columns have appeared in national and international magazines and newspapers, and in her book, *Room to Grow* (Norlights Press, 2009). Yoga, meditation, running, baking, writing, her work, family, and friendships light her world.

B.J. Dilley is an author and blogger living in Idaho with her husband and two children. She graduated from Arizona State University's Walter Cronkite School of Journalism, with honors, and has published two novels.

Kris Dinnison spent nearly two decades as a teacher and librarian. Her work has appeared in *One Teen Story*, *YARN*, *Germ Magazine*, HelloGiggles, among others. Her first novel, *You and Me and Him*, was published by Houghton Mifflin Harcourt. Kris loves to hike, read, and binge watch TV shows.

L. Joy Douglas resides in northern Indiana with her husband, two dogs and several chickens. Her work was first published in 2008. As a freelance writer, she has sold stories to several major publications and is currently working on her fifth book. Other interests include photography, reading and gluten-free cooking.

Drema Drudge is an MFA in Creative Writing graduate of Spalding University and is agented by Lisa Gallagher. Drema and her husband Barry live in Indiana, where she is working on her second novel. They are the proud parents of Mia and Zack. Learn more about Drema at dremadrudge.wordpress.com or on Twitter @dremadrudge.

B. R. Dunkelman has worked as an X-ray tech and Realtor, but has always been a writer. She is married and has one son, who is in the Navy. Brenda enjoys her small farm and all things Italian. She writes mostly fiction from her home in Chino, CA. More writing projects are in the works!

Joanna Dylan lives in a peaceful seaside community in New England with her author husband and very mischievous cat. In addition to writing, she loves exploring unknown areas, photography and hiking. She is currently writing a romantic suspense novel. She lives each day with a sense of gratitude and faith.

Maura Edwards is currently pursuing her Ph.D. She loves writing, cats, plants, and dancing.

Rebecca Eicksteadt is a health educator, fitness instructor, and writer living in Wisconsin. She received her Bachelor of Arts degree from the University of Wisconsin–Madison. She enjoys running, reading, painting, and leading worship at her church.

Shawnelle Eliasen and her husband Lonny have been married for twenty-six years. They raise five sons in an old Victorian near the Illinois banks of the Mississippi River. She's contributed to many titles in the *Chicken Soup for the Soul* series, and you can follow her adventures at shawnellewrites.blogspot.com.

Elizabeth Farella is a proud graduate of Molloy College where she received her teaching degree. She earned a master's degree in Reading from Adelphi University. She has been happily married for twenty-eight years and has three lovely daughters who inspired her story for this publication. E-mail her at jeeec@aol.com.

Victoria Fedden is the author of the memoir *This Is Not My Beautiful Life*, and she's also a mom and an English teacher. She lives in Fort Lauderdale, FL with her family. For updates and inspiration visit her at facebook.com/victoriacfedden.

Melanie Flint is a mother of three and a Licensed Clinical Social Worker currently in private practice in Houston, TX. She enjoys time with her husband and family in nature, road trips and cooking. Professionally,

Melanie takes a special interest in women's issues and supporting parents through the wondrous and choppy waters of parenthood.

Martine Foreman is a speaker, writer, blogger, and ACE-certified health coach. She enjoys reading, kickboxing, sandwiches, and a great glass of wine. Every day Martine gives thanks for her crazy, happy life with her husband, two kids, and her sassy cat, Pepper. Her first book will be published in 2017.

Marianne Fosnow resides in South Carolina. She was thrilled and honored to have a story included in *Chicken Soup for the Soul: The Spirit of America.* She's an avid reader and also enjoys photography.

Beck Gambill loves people. She works full-time as a high school paraprofessional, and loves raising two special kids with her husband. If there was one thing she could tell each person she meets it would be —"you matter!" She writes about living with purpose on her blog, *Becoming a Woman of Influence,* at becomingawomanofinfluence. wordpress.com.

Every summer **James Gemmell** can be found long-distance hiking in Europe. His hobbies, apart from hiking and hiking, are painting, art history, playing guitar and writing. James is the proud father of two grown children who can not only beat him in discussions but also at chess.

Jessica Ghigliotti is a stay-at-home, homeschooling mother of three children (so far). She enjoys painting in acrylics and watercolors, and remodeling the family's old fixer-upper home. She hopes to begin studying in a few years to become a midwife, and is currently working to publish her first children's book.

Angela Williams Glenn is a teacher, wife, mom of three, author of *Moms, Monsters, Media & Margaritas*, previous contributor to the

Chicken Soup for the Soul series, as well as the author of numerous other articles and essays on balancing motherhood with life. Read more of her writing on her blog *Stepping into Motherhood*.

Carmella de los Angeles Guiol is a Floridian gardener, dancer, adventurer, photographer, and writer. She has traveled to five continents and has worked as an artisan baker, organic farmer, and yacht deck hand. You can often find her kayaking the Hillsborough River, but you can always find her at therestlesswriter.com.

Georgia A. Hubley retired after twenty years from the money world to write about her world. Her stories appear in various anthologies and magazines. Once the nest was empty, Georgia and her husband of thirty-eight years left Silicon Valley and relocated to the Nevada desert. Learn more at georgiahubley.com.

Stephanie Tolliver Hyman is a native of the Appalachian Mountains. She earned a master's degree in English in 2005 and was the 2012 recipient of the R.J. Reynolds Excellence in Teaching Award. She has a beautiful daughter, Harper, a loving husband, Cory, and two affectionate cats, Sookie and Remi.

Carole Johnston received her Bachelor of Arts degree in Business Communications from Brock University in 1999. She lives with her husband, son and daughter in Ontario, Canada. Carole works at a local college, and enjoys running, going to the gym and reading. She loves to write pieces that people can relate to.

Devon Kab currently resides in Brooklyn, NY and works in Pharmaceutical Advertising/Plus Modeling. In her spare time Devon enjoys playing basketball and soccer, traveling, and speaking to the younger generation about positive body image. She became involved in modeling to share her journey of body confidence and self-love. E-mail her at devonkab@gmail.com.

Shannon Kaiser has been named in "100 Women to Watch in Wellness" by MindBodyGreen, and is a seven-time contributor to the *Chicken Soup for the Soul* series. She is the best-selling author of *Adventures for Your Soul* and the forthcoming book *The Self-Love Experiment* (August 2017). Connect with her on playwiththeworld.com.

Wendy Keppley, a Florida native, counseled troubled teens and taught college courses for high school honor students. She enjoys family, playing with her grandsons, and living in the woods near Tampa, FL. Wendy also loves writing, kayaking, reading, yoga, exploring waterfalls, and oneirology. E-mail her at wendykep@gmail.com.

Shelby Kisgen is a writer seeking publication for her debut novel. Her Bachelor of Arts degree qualifies her to work in many boring, entry-level positions. Instead, she follows her passion for stories. Shelby enjoys reading, traveling, and laughing with her husband.

Annie Kontor is a native Nebraskan and holds an M.A. degree from The University of Kansas. In true superhero fashion, she is a government employee by day and a freelance writer and editor at night. She is also the content creator of the PlusOneWoman.com blog, the only website geared specifically to single, curvy women.

Mallory Lavoie received her Bachelor of Arts degree from the University of Maine in 2012. She lives in Maine, where she works as a marketer and figure skating coach. She enjoys running, reading, playing the piano, and spending time with her dog, Mowgli.

After beating stage 3 endometrial cancer, **Kathryn Lehan** has reimagined her life helping other women learn how to use God's word to beat cancer and other chronic diseases. The ultimate goal of her company, Be Fruitful Alliance, is to teach women to unleash their divine purpose as an unstoppable warrior for Christ.

Alexes Lilly is a Toronto-based writer. She lives alone with two cats and a vivid imagination.

Maighread MacKay is the pen name of Margaret Hefferman, a Canadian author and visual artist from Durham Region in Ontario. She is a member of The Writers' Community of Durham Region (WCDR), the VFA (Visionary Fiction Alliance) and SINC (Sisters in Crime)–Toronto Chapter.

Debra Mayhew is a pastor's wife, mom to seven (usually) wonderful children, part-time teacher, editor and writer. She loves small town living, time with family, good books and long walks. Learn more at debramayhew.com.

Patrick Michael McIntyre graduated from James Lick High School in San Jose, CA in 1975. He is a father of two, stepfather to two more, as well as a proud grandparent of four. Michael, as he was called by SweetestRedHead, enjoys playing old-timers baseball, golf, and is currently writing a supernatural fictional work.

Phyllis McKinley cherishes life and finds something beautiful to admire each day. A former Canadian now living in Florida, she translates her common daily experiences into thoughtful poems and stories that have won many awards. This is her fifth contribution to the *Chicken Soup for the Soul* series. E-mail her at leafybough@hotmail.com.

Anne Merrigan is a therapist by trade, working in the field of trauma. Her personal experiences on "earth school" motivate her to assist others in discovering their own inner light. Anne enjoys painting, gardening, friends and family. E-mail her at creative13us@yahoo.com.

Jamie Leigh Miller received a Bachelor of Arts degree in Journalism from Southern Methodist University. She lives in Dallas, TX with her husband and pets. Jamie Leigh finds joy in sharing the tragically humorous moments in life with others.

Marya Morin is a freelance writer. Her stories and poems have appeared in publications such as *Woman's World* and Hallmark. Marya also penned a weekly humorous column for an online newsletter, and writes custom poetry on request. She lives in the country with her husband. E-mail her at Akushla514@hotmail.com.

Courtney Lynn Mroch is the Ambassador of Dark and Paranormal Tourism for Haunt Jaunts, a travel site for restless spirits. When she's not exploring haunted places or writing, it's a safe bet you'll find her on a tennis court or yoga mat somewhere. She lives in Nashville, TN with her husband.

Tamara Paylor is Associate Editor of *Daily Venus Diva* magazine, a plus lifestyle magazine; owns her own graphic and web design firm, Mae Lea Designs; and launched a clothing line as of January 2016 called Entrepreneur Life Apparel. Tamara enjoys being a mom and helping others become successful in business.

Beth Pugh is a wife, mother, and daughter trying to find contentment in a world of chaos. She writes hoping to inspire others to do the same by sharing lessons she's learned along the way. Her work has been published by The Good Men Project, Scary Mommy, *Sasee*, and *The Sun* magazine. E-mail her at bethiebug77@gmail.com.

Robin R. believes when inspiration strikes, you must act on it. When she's not acting on her latest inspiration, she can be found listening to classic rock music, blogging and playing with Samson (German Shepherd), Delilah (rescue), Sadie (Vizsla), Sable (Vizsla), and Sasha (rescue). Follow her on Twitter @RobinDarling.

Mudita Raj lives in Noida, India with her family. She is a student of Banasthali Vidyapeeth and is pursuing a B.A. degree. She is currently studying management, public administration and psychology. Mudita loves reading and watching movies.

Sunil Ramchandani is a fashion expert and creative director working with leading design firms in New York City. A graduate of FIT, he shares his love of style and design through his website and blog at sunilr.com.

Denise Reich is an Italian-born, New York–raised American-European freelance writer and lifelong *Star Wars* fan. She's a frequent contributor to the Canadian magazine *Shameless* and TheMighty.com. Her Broadway memoir, *Front of House*, was released in 2015.

J. Renee received her Doctor of Education Leadership degree from Harvard University and has devoted over fifteen years to working on behalf of children. She enjoys writing, public speaking, trying new recipes, and going for power walks. She is a member of the American Christian Fiction Writers. Learn more at jrenee.net.

Donna Roberts is a native upstate New Yorker who lives and works in Europe. She is an Associate Professor and holds a Ph.D. in Psychology. Donna is an animal and human rights advocate. When she is researching or writing, she can be found at her computer buried in rescue cats.

Jennifer Roberts writes under the pen names Jenna Mattison and JR Mattison. She is a filmmaker and novelist with her work displayed at The Academy of Motion Pictures Library and is also a best-selling mystery series author. Her movies have garnered international release and critical acclaim.

Regina Sunshine Robinson is a motivational speaker, talk show host and empowerment coach who wants to get you into a powerful "Regina Sunshine State of Mind"! Regina Sunshine loves sharing her message of self-love, positivity, and empowerment. Her motto is "It's Not Over Til I Win" and she wins when she sees others winning.

Lauren B. H. Rossato lives in Silver Spring, MD with an extensive collection of games and books, as well as a very tolerant husband. She may or may not have an addiction to yarn. Until this publication, her father did not know she was once an art model — Hi Dad!

Jillian Rossi is an author of horror, supernatural/science fiction and fantasy. She is a registered nurse and a member of the AACN. She advocates for pediatric oncology non-profit organizations to bring awareness to under-funding in development of better treatments. She currently lives in the South Bay with her family and son.

John Scanlan is a 1983 graduate of the United States Naval Academy, and retired from the Marine Corps as a Lieutenant Colonel aviator. He currently resides on Hilton Head Island, SC and is pursuing a second career as a writer. E-mail John at ping1@hargray.com.

Jenni Schaefer is a National Recovery Advocate with Eating Recovery Center (ERC, 877-957-6575). ERC provides specialized eating disorders treatment across the U.S. ERC's Insight Behavioral Health Centers (877-737-7391) provide treatment for mood and anxiety disorders, including PTSD. Learn more at JenniSchaefer.com/Seek-Help.

Jenna Schifferle earned a bachelor's degree from State University of New York at Oswego, where she graduated *summa cum laude*, and a master's degree from the University of Rochester. She hangs her heart in Buffalo, NY, but keeps her running sneakers ready to hop on the first flight going anywhere. Learn more at Jenna.Schifferle.wordpress.com.

Sherri Shepherd is an Emmy Award winner as co-host on the hit ABC talk show *The View*. She executive produced and created her own sitcom, *Sherri*, on Lifetime television. She is a New York Times best-selling author for her book *Plan D: How to Lose Weight and Beat Diabetes Even if You Don't Have To*. Sherri can be seen co-staring alongside John Lithgow in the new NBC comedy *Trial & Error* starting March 2017. Sherri has a beautiful son Jeffrey and two dogs, Lexi and Ashley.

Danielle Sibila was born in Southern California and moved to North Alabama after high school. She enjoys creating and fixing anything, from knitting to heavy equipment maintenance. She would like to acknowledge her friends and family, for their innumerable contributions in her life.

Ashley M. Slayton is an award-winning blogger and multimedia journalist. Ashley has written for BET.com, *002houston*, *D CEO*, the *Longview News-Journal* and the *Daily American*. She currently works as a digital producer for KLTV 7.

Kelly Smith is a writer and changer of diapers who believes that people are essentially good. She lives with her husband and sons in the Midwest where she is a college communications instructor. Kelly earned her master's degree in English from Northern Illinois University and recently completed writing her first novel.

Jennifer Sommerfelt lives in Iowa with her husband and three daughters with whom she loves to dance. She would like to thank her friend and old college roommate, Jennifer Rathe, for writing her story in such a fun and creative way to inspire others. Jennifer is happy to be a part of the beginning of her friend's writing career.

Diane Stark is a wife, mother of five, former teacher, and freelance writer. She loves to write about the important things in life: her family and her faith. E-mail her at DianeStark19@yahoo.com.

L.A. Strucke is a freelance writer from New Jersey and earned her Bachelor of Arts degree from Rowan University. She is a frequent contributor to the *Chicken Soup for the Soul* series, *Guideposts* and other publications. A mother of four, she enjoys writing about family and inspirational pieces. Read more at lastrucke.com.

Jimmie Ware is a freelance writer and poetess. She has lived in Chicago, Alabama, Alaska and currently resides in Arizona with her daughter Nicole where they continue to perform and host poetry events. Jimmie is founder of the Black Feather Poets and former radio personality on KFAT 92.9FM in Anchorage. Jimmie breathes poetry.

Dorann Weber has been a fan of *Chicken Soup for the Soul* books since they were first published in 1993. She loved them so much she tried her hand at writing stories. She is a freelance photographer for a local newspaper and a Getty Images contributor. She lives in New Jersey with her family. E-mail her at dorann_weber@yahoo.com.

Jenny Wildflower is the owner of Wildflower Floral Events, a successful wedding and event floral design company in the Hamptons. She is also the proud mother of a USMC veteran. Her flowers are made in an 1800's old barn located behind her yellow farmhouse.

Following a fifteen-year career in nuclear medicine, **Melissa Wootan** is joyfully exploring her creative side. She enjoys refurbishing old furniture but is most passionate about writing. Her stories have appeared in the *Chicken Soup for the Soul* series and *Guideposts*. Contact her at facebook.com/chicvintique.

A. Kay Wyatt writes from her home city of Chicago, IL. Along with writing, she explores the city on skateboard, plays guitar, and tends bar. On the weekends, she coaches high school students in the art of rhetorical debate. She lives with her cat, Dr. Indiana Bones.

Brenda Yoder is a licensed Mental Health Counselor, Life Coach, writer and motivational speaker on life, faith, and parenting beyond the storybook image. She is a wife and mom to four kids, teens to adults, and lives on a farm in Indiana.

Maxine Young is a writer based in New York City. She is an avid listener of audiobooks, a passionate lover of tea and an enduring fighter of multiple sclerosis. She is a big fan of planting seeds of encouragement. E-mail her at maxiney7@gmail.com.

Lydia Young-Samson has a Master's of Education, and taught science for four years before becoming a full-time author and starting her own business. Her blog and devotional can be found at theunculturedchristian. wordpress.com. She is currently working on her first fiction book and is getting settled in her marriage.

Lori Zenker likes to walk and talk (even in snowstorms) around the small Ontario, Canada town she lives in. She's a mom of three teenagers and collects and sells old junk. She loves to write, and is always on the hunt for inspiration to write — this is the sixth *Chicken Soup for the Soul* book she's been privileged to be a part of.

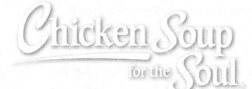

Meet Amy Newmark

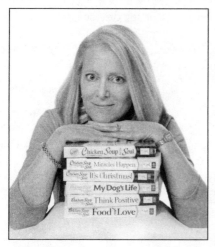

Amy Newmark is the bestselling author, editor-in-chief, and publisher of the *Chicken Soup for the Soul* book series. Since 2008, she has published 135 new books, most of them national bestsellers in the U.S. and Canada, more than doubling the number of Chicken Soup for the Soul titles in print today. She is also the author of *Simply Happy*, a crash course in Chicken Soup for the Soul advice and wisdom that is filled with easy-to-implement, practical tips for having a better life.

Amy is credited with revitalizing the Chicken Soup for the Soul brand, which has been a publishing industry phenomenon since the first book came out in 1993. By compiling inspirational and aspirational true stories curated from ordinary people who have had extraordinary experiences, Amy has kept the twenty-three-year-old Chicken Soup for the Soul brand fresh and relevant.

Amy graduated *magna cum laude* from Harvard University where she majored in Portuguese and minored in French. She then embarked on a three-decade career as a Wall Street analyst, a hedge fund manager, and a corporate executive in the technology field. She is a Chartered Financial Analyst.

Her return to literary pursuits was inevitable, as her honors thesis in college involved traveling throughout Brazil's impoverished northeast region, collecting stories from regular people. She is delighted to have come full circle in her writing career — from collecting stories "from the people" in Brazil as a twenty-year-old to, three decades later, collecting stories "from the people" for Chicken Soup for the Soul.

When Amy and her husband Bill, the CEO of Chicken Soup for the Soul, are not working, they are visiting their four grown children.

Follow Amy on Twitter and Instagram @amynewmark. Listen to her free daily podcast, The Chicken Soup for the Soul Podcast, at www.chickensoup.podbean.com, or find it on iTunes, the Podcasts app on iPhone, or on your favorite podcast app on other devices.

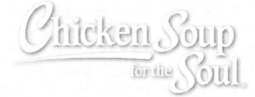

Meet Supermodel Emme

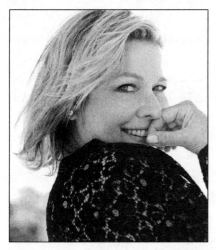

For over two decades as a leading voice and face in the fashion industry, Emme is the iconic world's first curvy supermodel. With the conviction that beauty comes in all shapes and sizes, Emme has paved the way and given women the platform to feel beautiful and empowered.

A TV personality, model, mom, author, brand spokesperson, creative director of her clothing lines, lecturer and globally recognized women's advocate for positive body image and self-esteem, Emme's message is clear — *to awaken the inner magnificence inherent in each of us, to be whole.*

Emme is often consulted and interviewed in the media on eating disorders and body image, fashion trends and model diversity, as well as surviving cancer and women's health. She has appeared on all the major networks, including on *Today, Good Morning America, CBS The Early Show,* CNN, MSNBC, *Access Hollywood,* and *Entertainment Tonight.* Her press coverage includes *The New York Times, Women's Wear Daily, People, Glamour, Marie Claire, TIME,* and the *Wall Street Journal.*

She has twice been selected to *People Magazine's* "50 Most Beautiful People" and *Ladies' Home Journal* chose her as one of the "Most Important

Women in America" and one of the "Most Fascinating Women of the Year." These accolades are truly representative of her tireless commitment to advocacy. She has also been honored as one of *Glamour* magazine's "Women of the Year" and as one of *Biography* magazine's "25 Most Influential Women." Emme is an ambassador to The National Eating Disorders Association, honorary board member to Project Heal, and also donates her time to the Girl Scouts of America.

Emme's passion for nature and fitness fuels her active lifestyle, which includes snowshoeing, boogie boarding, bike-athons, hiking, yoga and swimming.

Emme's podcast — EMME: Life Lessons — is available at www. letscabana.com.

Emme's new activewear and athleisure line is available on www. EmmeSport.com.

Emme's ongoing inclusive fashion design initiative — Fashion Without Limits: Changing the Face of Fashion — teaches future fashion designers in design school how to design for a full size range of women, size 0-24. For more information on it, please visit www. FashionWithoutLimits.org.

To learn more and sign up for Emme's newsletter please go to www. emmestyle.com; follow her on social media at @SupermodelEmme.

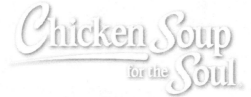

Meet Natasha Stoynoff

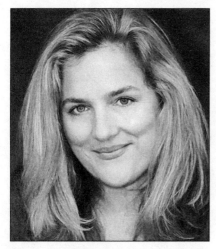

Natasha Stoynoff began her career as a teenaged entertainment sleuth in her hometown of Toronto, nabbing interviews and photos of elusive celebrities like Bruce Springsteen, Marlon Brando, and Madonna for the local dailies.

After earning a B.A. in English and Psychology at York University and studying Journalism, she worked as a two-way news reporter/photographer at the *Toronto Star* and created her own Showbiz column, "Celebrity Bytes," at the *Toronto Sun*.

While still in Canada, Natasha became a correspondent for *People* and *TIME* magazines, covering the Cannes International Film Festival and reporting for cover stories on sports, politics, and human interest. Before the turn of the century, she moved to New York City to join *People* on staff, where she remained for more than a decade interviewing top film and music icons including Meryl Streep, Paul McCartney, and Lauren Bacall.

This is her twelfth book collaboration, including two New York Times bestsellers. Natasha lives in Manhattan, where she works on screenplays and books.

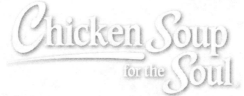

Thank You

We are grateful to all our contributors and fans, who shared their stories about the most personal topics imaginable — their body image, self-esteem, and appearance. We had thousands of submissions and they all had an impact on the final book, informing us as to what's on the minds of women, and a few men, today, regarding this important topic. Barbara LoMonaco, Kristiana Pastir, and D'ette Corona were our readers, and they narrowed down the list to a few hundred finalists for Emme, Natasha, and Amy to consider.

Associate Publisher D'ette Corona continued to be Amy's right-hand woman in creating the final manuscript and working with all our wonderful writers. Barbara LoMonaco and Kristiana Pastir, along with outside proofreader Elaine Kimbler, jumped in at the end to proof, proof, proof. And yes, there will always be typos anyway, so feel free to let us know about them at webmaster@chickensoupforthesoul.com and we will correct them in future printings.

The whole publishing team deserves a hand, including Senior Director of Marketing Maureen Peltier, Executive Assistant Mary Fisher, Senior Director of Production Victor Cataldo, Editor Ronelle Frankel and graphic designer Daniel Zaccari, who turned our manuscript into this beautiful book.

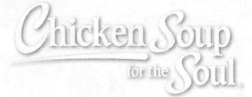

Sharing Happiness, Inspiration, and Hope

Real people sharing real stories, every day, all over the world. In 2007, *USA Today* named *Chicken Soup for the Soul* one of the five most memorable books in the last quarter-century. With over 100 million books sold to date in the U.S. and Canada alone, more than 200 titles in print, and translations into more than forty languages, "chicken soup for the soul" is one of the world's best-known phrases.

Today, twenty-three years after we first began sharing happiness, inspiration and hope through our books, we continue to delight our readers with new titles, but have also evolved beyond the bookstore, with super premium pet food and a variety of licensed products and digital offerings, all inspired by stories. Chicken Soup for the Soul has recently expanded into visual storytelling through movies and television. Chicken Soup for the Soul is "changing the world one story at a time®." Thanks for reading!

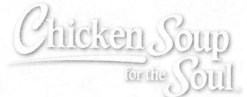

Share with Us

We all have had Chicken Soup for the Soul moments in our lives. If you would like to share your story or poem with millions of people around the world, go to chickensoup.com and click on "Submit Your Story." You may be able to help another reader and become a published author at the same time. Some of our past contributors have launched writing and speaking careers from the publication of their stories in our books!

We only accept story submissions via our website. They are no longer accepted via mail or fax.

To contact us regarding other matters, please send us an e-mail through webmaster@chickensoupforthesoul.com, or fax or write us at:

Chicken Soup for the Soul
P.O. Box 700
Cos Cob, CT 06807-0700
Fax: 203-861-7194

One more note from your friends at Chicken Soup for the Soul: Occasionally, we receive an unsolicited book manuscript from one of our readers, and we would like to respectfully inform you that we do not accept unsolicited manuscripts and we must discard the ones that appear.

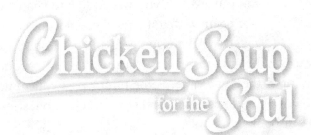

Changing your life one story at a time®
www.chickensoup.com